VITAMIN DISCOVERIES
AND DISASTERS

VITAMIN DISCOVERIES AND DISASTERS

History, Science, and Controversies

FRANCES RACHEL FRANKENBURG, M.D.

The Praeger Series on Contemporary Health and Living

PRAEGER
An Imprint of ABC-CLIO, LLC

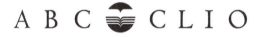

A B C CLIO

Santa Barbara, California • Denver, Colorado • Oxford, England

Library of Congress Cataloging-in-Publication Data

Frankenburg, Frances Rachel.
    Vitamin discoveries and disasters : history, science, and controversies /
Frances Rachel Frankenburg.
        p. ; cm. — (Praeger series on contemporary health and living)
    Includes bibliographical references and index.
        ISBN 978-0-313-35475-5 (hard copy : alk. paper)—978-0-313-35476-2 (ebook)
        1. Vitamins—History. 2. Vitamins in human nutrition—History.
3. Avitaminosis—History. I. Title. II. Series: Praeger series on contemporary
health and living.
        [DNLM: 1. Vitamins—history. 2. Avitaminosis—history. 3. Research—history.
4. Research Personnel—Biography. QU 11.1 F829v 2009]

QP771.F73   2009
612.3′99—dc22   2009011021

13   12   11   10   9   1   2   3   4   5

This book is also available on the World Wide Web as an ebook.
Visit www.abc-clio.com for details.

ABC-CLIO, LLC
130 Cremona Drive, P.O. Box 1911
Santa Barbara, California 93116-1911

This book is printed on acid-free paper ∞

Manufactured in the United States of America

CONTENTS

Contents

Series Foreword

Contemporary Health and Living

Over the past one hundred years, there have been incredible medical break-throughs that have prevented or cured illness in billions of people and helped many more improve their health while living with chronic conditions. A few of the most important twentieth-century discoveries include antibiotics, organ transplants, and vaccines. The twenty-first century has already heralded important new treatments, including such things as a vaccine to prevent human papillomavirus from infecting and potentially leading to cervical cancer in women. Polio is on the verge of being eradicated worldwide, making it only the second infectious disease behind smallpox to ever be erased as a human health threat.

In this series, experts from many disciplines share with readers important and updated medical knowledge. All aspects of health are considered, including subjects that are disease specific and preventive medical care. Disseminating this information will help individuals to improve their health, researchers to determine where there are gaps in our current knowledge, and policy-makers to assess the most pressing needs in healthcare.

Series Editor Julie K. Silver, M.D.
Assistant Professor
Harvard Medical School
Department of Physical Medicine and Rehabilitation

Acknowledgments

I am grateful to the following people who have been generous in their help: Ross J. Baldessarini, Ruth Becker, Sanford Becker, Gregory Binus, Eve Camerman, Debbie Carvalko, Ian Cohen, Gary Cole, Lucy Cole, Charles Drebing, Charles Frankenburg, Dennis Frankenburg, Naomi Frankenburg, Robert Frankenburg, Susi Frankenburg, Michelle Gelfand, Elizabeth Grynberg, Diane Hartwell, Ana Ivkovic, Odie Kaplan, Shannon LeMaster, Joan Margeson, Honey Maser, John Riley, Ethan Rofman, Ken Silk, Julie Silver Al Sommer, Linda Tenenbaum, Catherine Zahn, Jeff Zahn, and Mary Zanarini.

Introduction

We all know that we should eat a variety of foods, including dairy products and fresh fruits and vegetables, because these foods contain vitamins. This is so obvious that it hardly bears repeating, yet the discoveries of vitamins involve stories of adventure and heroism that are not well known. It is difficult today to realize how much courage and perseverance the scientists who discovered vitamins possessed.

Researchers in the 1800s believed that they could "make" food in the laboratory by mixing up the right combinations of fats, carbohydrates, proteins, water, and minerals. It seemed that nutrition had been mastered. Moreover, scientists were just discovering that bacteria caused illnesses. What could diet possibly have to do with illness? However, people and laboratory animals eating artificial diets did not survive. Plants, bacteria, and fungi make complicated molecules that are different from fats, carbohydrates, or proteins and could not easily be made in the laboratory. These products, which we need in very small quantities, are vitamins. Each vitamin has an irreplaceable role in the body's metabolism. Without vitamins, diseases such as scurvy and beriberi develop.

Investigations into these vitamin deficiency diseases were not simple. This was more than painstaking chemical work in a laboratory, although it was that too. The scientists involved often worked in dreadful circumstances and almost always had to face the ridicule of their colleagues, including the infectious disease specialists of the day. Some of these scientists, such as Edward Vedder, Albert Hess, and Robert Williams, refused to accept the inevitability of human suffering and were relentless in their pursuit of cures for illnesses. In this book, we will review the stories of these and other scientists and explain how vitamins, which today we take for granted, were discovered.

Some scientists had to work in secret. For example, in 1907, Elmer McCollum, a scientist from Kansas, and Marguerite Davis set up the first American rat colonies in Madison, Wisconsin. This was done in a clandestine manner because the dean of the agricultural college at Wisconsin disapproved of experiments with rats. Their work led to the discovery of Vitamin A, or retinol.

Some scientists worked for decades, and some scientists had moments of insight. For example, Christiaan Eijkman was investigating the epidemic of beriberi in Indonesia. People with "dry" beriberi suffered from severe pains in their legs, making it impossible for them to walk. People with "wet" beriberi had heart disease, leading to swollen legs. Eijkman saw ill Indochinese chickens staggering around his compound and, in a flash of genius, noted the resemblance to beriberi and traced this to a change in their diet. This realization that a change in the diet could cause illness was a pivotal moment in the history of human health.

Eijkman was mocked for this insight, as was Joseph Goldberger, another inventive and persistent man. In 1914, the U.S. Public Health Services sent Joseph Goldberger to the South, where pellagra was endemic, to find the microbe that caused pellagra. Goldberger, an expert in infectious diseases, suspected that there might be a nutritional component to the illness. He arranged an experiment on prisoners in Mississippi, in which their diet was deliberately manipulated to cause illness. This trial was successful but was criticized mercilessly by physicians of the South who continued to blame a microbe.

In one of the more personal experiments that will be described in this book, William Castle at Harvard gave some of his patients who were ill with pernicious anemia meat digested by his own stomach juices. He concluded from this experiment that two factors were involved in the successful liver therapy of pernicious anemia. The factor in his stomach juice turned out to be cobalamin. This is another example of an experiment that makes us feel a bit queasy, that would without a doubt not be allowed to happen today, and that helped us to understand how vitamins work.

In the past, children in industrial cities or northern latitudes developed soft bones that bowed out under their own weight. By the beginning of the twentieth century, scientists knew that this condition, rickets, was associated with faulty mineralization of bone and was somehow associated with poor diet or lack of exposure to sunlight. Harry Steenbock in Wisconsin, Alfred Hess in New York, and Harriette Chick in London, also known as the heroine of Vienna for her work in that post–World War I city, showed that rickets could be prevented by either sunlight or cod-liver oil, an unlikely pair of treatments. These scientists were able to work successfully with two very different approaches to this strange situation and discovered Vitamin D, or calcitriol. Vitamin D is not actually a vitamin, as long as we are exposed to sufficient sunlight. Even though Vitamin D is in some respects not a "real" vitamin, it is the one vitamin in which large numbers of Americans may be deficient.

Because of the courage, intelligence, and persistence of the scientists reviewed in this book, we understand far more about the elements needed for a healthy diet than we did a hundred years ago. This understanding, combined with technological advances in agriculture, food preservation, refrigeration, and transportation, has meant that vitamin deficiency diseases rarely occur in the developed world. The amazing stories of vitamin deficiencies of the past, and the discovery of their cures, are recounted in the following pages.

1

RATS THAT DON'T GROW AND HAVE SORE EYES: VITAMIN A (RETINOL), THE ANTI-NIGHT BLINDNESS VITAMIN

OVERVIEW

In the early 1900s an agricultural scientist established secret rat colonies in Wisconsin. This project led to a series of discoveries. One of the first was that newborn rats grew best when fed on diets containing some animal fats. Without butterfat or cod-liver oil in their diet, the rodents grew poorly, became ill with infections such as pneumonia, developed inflamed eyes, and were likely to die. Japanese and Danish physicians discovered that children also needed to eat these fats to grow normally and remain healthy. The important substance in these fats turned out to be Vitamin A. In 1932 an English physician successfully treated children ill with measles with Vitamin A. This is because the immune system, which protects us from infections, and the skin and lining of many organs and tissues, depend on Vitamin A.

Vitamin A also allows us to see in dim light and plays a role in the production of tears, which lubricate and moisten the eye. For many decades, most of the interest in Vitamin A centered on eye ailments, such as night blindness and dry eyes. People without enough of this vitamin develop eyes that are so dry and ulcerated that the cornea can burst, leading to total blindness. An ophthalmologist studying eye problems in Indonesian children in the 1970s discovered that Vitamin A deficiency was also associated with infections and deaths. This finding astonished most physicians of the time but would not have been a surprise to earlier scientists or physicians.

Testing for Butterfat at the University of Wisconsin

Many discoveries in human nutrition came from research done in agricultural and veterinary laboratories. Much work was done at the University of Wisconsin, which had as one of its missions the improvement of the quality of cows and dairy products. Stephen Babcock (1843–1931), one of the great agricultural chemists from this university, grew up on a farm in Oneida, in upstate New York. He studied chemistry at Tufts and Cornell. In the 1870s he went to Germany to study with pupils of Justus von Liebig (1803–1873). Liebig and his students had introduced new methods to the field of nutrition. They turned it into a quantitative science and used laboratory apparatus to calculate the exact percentages of protein, fat, carbohydrate, salt, and water that were needed in diets. This work supported the hope of some scientists: the liberation of our nutrition from actual food. In later years, Babcock would veer sharply from these interests.

ARTIFICIAL FOOD

Food made in the laboratory promised to free people from depending on natural foods. It proved more difficult to reproduce foods in the laboratory than hoped. There were some famous catastrophic experiments. For example, in 1816, François Magendie (1783–1855) fed dogs on sugar and water. Their eyes dried out, ulcerated, and burst.

During a war between France and Germany in 1870, Paris was under siege, and its citizens, especially children, were starving. Milk and eggs were unavailable. A chemist prepared artificial milk by mixing fat in a sweet solution, but to no avail. Children died.

We now know that these artificial foods could not sustain life because of their inadequate protein and vitamin content.

Babcock received a doctorate in organic chemistry at the University of Göttingen and returned to the United States to work at the Geneva Experimental Station in New York. In 1888, he moved to the University of Wisconsin, where his first task was to solve a vexing problem for dairy farmers. The farmers were not able to sell their customers milk of consistent quality. The quality of milk depended in part on the amount of butterfat in the milk. Milk was sometimes watered down because the farmers were paid for the quantity, not the quality, of the milk. Customers never quite knew the quality of milk that they were buying. This was not helpful for the industry because it cast a shadow on all dairymen and their products.

Throughout the 1880s, many scientists around the world were working on the same problem: how to devise a simple and accurate way of measuring the amount of butterfat in milk. Babcock devised a simple method of doing this. He took a sample of milk and added sulfuric acid to it, which dissolved everything except the butterfat. He spun the milk sample in a calibrated bottle in a centrifuge or rotor-type machine, and the fat rose to the top. The fat layer in the centrifuged milk could then be easily measured. Milk became a more consistent product. Consumers knew what they were buying. Dairy farmers used this test to determine which of their cows or which type of feed yielded milk with the highest concentration of butterfat.

Babcock never patented this invention, believing that it belonged to the public. He later regretted this decision. By not patenting it, he lost control of

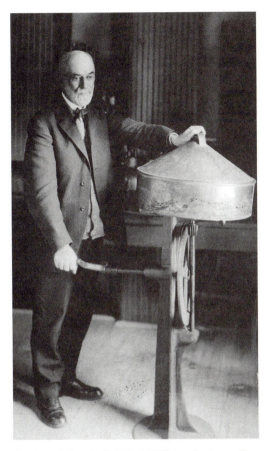

Stephen Babcock (1843–1931) is spinning milk
in a centrifuge in order that its butterfat, which
contains Vitamin A, can be measured. This picture
is from about 1925. Courtesy University of
Wisconsin–Madison Archives.

the device that bore his name. Other manufacturers produced inferior testing
equipment that produced faulty "Babcock tests." This decision would influence Harry Steenbock some years later in his work with Vitamin D.

Single-Grain Experiment

Babcock moved on to his next task. He wondered whether, in determining
the protein, fat, carbohydrate, salt, and water content of diets, and nothing
else, Liebig had missed something. Dairy farmers believed that cows did best
when grazing on a number of different plants, and Babcock thought that the
farmers might have known something that was not captured in the laboratories of Göttingen.

In 1907 Babcock arranged an experiment to check Liebig's theory. This became known as the "single-grain experiment." He devised four different feeding plans for sixteen heifers, all five months old:

- corn only;
- wheat only;
- oats only; or
- a mixture of the three grains.

All diets were manipulated to contain the same amount of protein, fat, carbohydrate, salt, and water. According to what he had learned in Göttingen, all of the heifers should have grown at the same rate. For the first year or so, this seemed to be the case. They grew well, and there was little difference between them. He bred the cows. The experiment then became more interesting. The calves of the corn-fed cows were healthy, but the calves of the other three groups were less healthy. Over the next few months all of the cows, except those fed on just corn, became weak and ill. In 1909, some of the cows fed on wheat alone died. A young scientist, E. V. McCollum, described these cows:

> They presented amazing contrasts. The wheat-fed cows were small of girth and rough-coated. They were all blind, as shown by the lead color of the eyes and by their inability to find their way about. Each had recently given birth to a greatly undersized premature calf and all calves were dead when born. The oat-fed cows carried their young to full term. Though the calves were of normal weight at birth, all but one were dead then . . . The corn-fed cows were, by standards of animal husbandry, in excellent condition . . . Though all the cows had had feed of the same chemical composition, they differed enormously. . . .[1]

Babcock and his team never succeeded in fully understanding these dramatic and unexpected findings, but the experiment was important in that it pointed to the great gaps in knowledge of nutrition. According to the theories of the day, the cows should have all done equally well. All of the measurements and chemical analyses in laboratories could not explain the decline in the cows fed on wheat, or oats, or the mix of three grains. Food contained more than Liebig's chemical components. This study also showed that it was important to study animals throughout their life cycle. Brief studies were not helpful.

"Accessory Factors" in England and Vermin in Wisconsin

Biochemists in Europe were also beginning to break away from the idea that the only factors in food that mattered were the proteins, carbohydrates, and fats. At the beginning of the twentieth century, the British biochemist Sir Frederick Gowland Hopkins (1861–1947) established one of the world's great biochemical research institutions at Cambridge. He showed in experiments with mice and rats that foods contained other substances that were important for nutrition. For example, rats (and humans) cannot make all of the amino acids, the building blocks that make up proteins, and need to have "essential amino acids" in the diet. Hopkins discovered tryptophan in 1901. This will be discussed further in the chapter about Vitamin B3. Hopkins was revered for the encouragement he gave to many younger scientists. An eminent man, he was known to all as "Hoppy."

In a lecture in 1912, Hopkins explained that these substances were "accessory factors" because they were needed in *addition* to proteins, carbohydrates, fats, salt, and water. He was also one of the first people to describe the nutritional benefits of yeast extracts. Would observations like those of Hopkins in England be of any value for farmers raising cows and pigs in Wisconsin? Many people thought not. The dean of the agricultural college at Wisconsin was not impressed by experiments with rats, and he had no interest in supporting similar work at his college. Farmers in Wisconsin wanted their tax dollars going to exterminate vermin, not to house and feed them.

Dr. Vitamin, Secret Studies, Rats, and Fats

The scientist who convinced the University of Wisconsin that it was time to think smaller was the young man who had described the cows in the single-grain experiment. Elmer Verner McCollum (1879–1967) was born to homesteaders in Kansas. As a child he helped to raise pigs and saw that they grew better when supplied with ample amounts of milk. He trapped and killed rats, for which he was paid a bounty. As an adult he would return to these interests and activities. He was originally interested in medicine, but became enchanted by organic chemistry. He attended Yale, where he received a Ph.D. in chemistry. In 1907 he accepted a position at Wisconsin, where he was part of the single-grain experiment team. His role was to analyze the food and feces from Babcock's cows.

McCollum worked with large quantities of foodstuff and dung. He became discouraged by this work. He ended up thinking that the wheat-fed cows did so badly because there was no "green leaf" included in their feed and that the experiment perhaps had not been planned very carefully. He wrote, "Through four years we had been inexcusably uncritical of some important details."[2] Perhaps not surprisingly, he came to appreciate the value of smaller animals. He decided to work with rats. He did this in secret at first because of the dean's opposition. He began by using wild barn rats. Once again, he was trapping rats, using the same techniques he used as a child, but now to use in experiments. The barn rats were savage and unmanageable. He realized that his work would be easier if the rats were tame so he bought white, or albino, rats from a pet shop. These rats were cheap, hardy, and easy to house, handle, and feed. Experiments done on rats, rather than cows, had the following advantages:

- They could be conducted in smaller spaces, with less food, and on hundreds of animals at a time.
- Results could be gathered more quickly because the life span of a rat is shorter than the life span of a cow.
- Female rats bear litters with multiple babies at three months of age, so it was possible to maintain a large supply of experimental animals.

McCollum and his colleague Marguerite Davis set up the first American rat colonies in Wisconsin in 1907. They set up a long series of experiments in which they fed rats carefully measured diets. They added components one by one, which allowed them to be certain of the effects of each component. He was determined, in this set of experiments, to pay attention to the "important details" that had been missed in earlier work.

McCollum was at the mercy of the albino rodents. If they did not cooperate with him, he might have had to return to cow dung. McCollum and Davis investigated the possibility that some of the diets fed to the rats were not palatable—the rats would not eat the food. Rats, like humans, had food preferences and turned up their snouts at bland repetitive diets. They tried to make the diets appealing to the rats by adding strong flavors, such as cheese extracts, bacon, or cinnamon. As always, the value of the experiments depended on the care taken in all aspects of the work. Despite this great care, we shall read in the scurvy chapter that at one point in his work with laboratory animals, McCollum underestimated the importance of ensuring that the animals ate what the technicians wanted them to.

This work was difficult and confusing, although physically easier than examining cow dung. Other universities also began to work with rats, but different labs and colonies could not find the same results. One problem turned out to be milk sugar, or lactose. Some researchers used milk sugar as a source of calories, without fully purifying it. Small amounts of milk protein, or fat, could supply the rats with amino acids or vitamins unbeknownst to the researchers. The researchers were not aware for some time that minute quantities of substances, which turned out to be vitamins, were essential for health.

Another problem was rat feces. Rats often eat their own droppings and the droppings of their cage mates, and this complicated any nutritional experiments because droppings often contain vitamins. If the researchers did not take this into account, they did not always know what their rats were eating. Unappealing as it is, this is not the only occasion in which coprophagia, the eating of feces, is mentioned. Coprophagia can be healthy. Feces and vitamins will be discussed again in the chapters about Vitamins B9, B12, and D.

McCollum and Davis persevered. They recorded every element of their rats' growth and wellness and made a series of discoveries after some years of frustration. One of the first discoveries to come out of the Wisconsin rat colonies had to do with fats. Liebig and others had shown that fat was an essential nutrient. The German workers thought that fat was only needed for energy and that all fats were the same. McCollum used different fats and recorded the rats' responses to each fat. The idea that there were nutritional consequences to different kinds of fats was new.

McCollum's pet rats grew well on diets where the fat came from butter, egg yolks, or cod-liver oil. The rodents did not grow well if the fat came from olive oil, lard, or almond oil. They developed sore eyes and often died from infections, such as pneumonia. In 1913, after much work with these various fats, the researchers found a substance in butter, egg, and cod-liver oil that was not present in the vegetable fats and that could be dissolved in other fats. This was the first vitamin to be identified, although the word vitamin was not then in use. As can be imagined, this discovery made the Wisconsin dairy farmers and the dean of the agricultural college happy. The colonies came out of hiding. Working with rats had led McCollum to prove the value of butter.

Sweet and Wholesome Butter Versus an Artificial Compound of Grease

For the rest of his life McCollum promoted the virtues of butter. In a book on nutrition that he and his wife wrote for the general public, he lauded this fat: "Butter tastes better than any other fat. It is the only fat which is elaborated by nature for the specific purpose of affording nourishment."[3]

McCollum shared these convictions with dairy farmers and their politicians who were fiercely protective of butter, especially when it came to competition with margarine. Margarine had many advantages over butter. It was cheaper, did not rely on the availability of fresh milk with ample butterfat, and did not turn rancid. This was particularly important in the days before refrigeration. In 1887 Governor Lucius Hubbard of Minnesota (a butter-producing state) said, in defense of butter and in opposition to margarine, "The public has been victim of various impositions practiced in different departments of its industry, but I think that it will be admitted that the ingenuity of depraved human genius has culminated in the production of oleomargarine and its kindred abominations."[4]

MARGARINE

In 1869 a French pharmacist, Hippolyte Mège-Mouriés, developed margarine in response to a contest organized by Napoleon III, who was looking for a cheap and artificial fat. Mège-Mouriés used animal fat and flavored it with a small amount of milk. Originally made from animal fat, margarine is now usually made with vegetable oils.

In Wisconsin margarine was treated as a dangerous chemical intruder. In 1902 Wisconsin Senator Joseph Quarles (1843–1911) reminded people that, in those days, margarine was made from chopped-up beef fat, or lard. He drew a passionate comparison between butter and margarine:

Things have come to a strange pass when the steer competes with the cow as a butter maker. When the hog conspires with the steer to monopolize the dairy business, it is time for self-respecting men to take up the cudgels for the cow . . . We ought not now to desert her or permit her to be displaced, her sweet and wholesome product supplanted by an artificial compound of grease that may be chemically pure but has never known the fragrance of clover, the

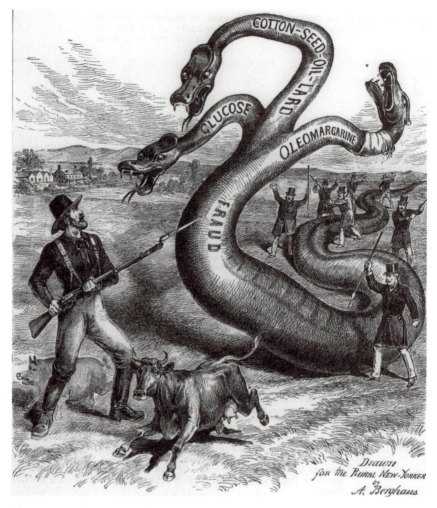

This cartoon shows a three-headed hydra, representing oleomargarine, threatening a
farmer. This was originally drawn for the *Rural New-Yorker* by A. Berghaus and
demonstrated the suspicion with which the introduction of margarine was greeted.
The listed ingredients of margarine—cotton seed oil, lard, and glucose—would not
have contained Vitamin A. Margarine is now fortified with Vitamin A. Wisconsin
Historical Society.

freshness of dew or the exquisite flavor which nature bestows exclusively on
butter fat to adapt it to the taste of man . . . I desire butter that comes from the
dairy, not the slaughterhouse. I want butter that has the natural aroma of life
and health. I decline to accept as a substitute caul fat, matured under the chill
of death, blended with vegetable oils and flavored by chemical tricks.[5]

McCollum and Davis: Fat-Soluble Factor A and Water-Soluble Factor B

McCollum and Davis were aware of the work of Casimir Funk, who had suggested the existence of substances called "vitamines." (This work is described in more detail in Chapter 2.) They knew that a diet of polished rice caused beriberi. In 1915 they formulated a clear hypothesis that the diet had to contain protein, a source of energy, salts, and at least two unidentified substances. Not liking the word "vitamine," they called the substance found in butterfat and cod-liver oil *fat-soluble factor A,* and the other substance found in plants *water-soluble factor B.* It was later discovered that there were other vitamins and that the *water-soluble factor B* was a large group of substances, but their 1915 hypothesis was clear and focused the young field of nutrition. Eventually, McCollum's *fat-soluble factor A* became known as Vitamin A.

McCollum Is Recruited by Johns Hopkins

In 1917 McCollum was recruited from the college of agriculture at the University of Wisconsin by the Johns Hopkins School of Hygiene and Public Health in Baltimore. This was an unusual recruitment. And so it seemed to McCollum himself. In his autobiography, he wrote, "Out of a clear sky I had been appointed to a professorship in the most notable research university in the country . . . I could scarcely realize that I, a worker in an agricultural experiment station, with no medical training and no contacts with public health, was the first professor selected to take charge of a department in the new and exciting adventure of training medical and nonmedical students. . . ."[6]

In making this appointment, Johns Hopkins was taking the unusual step of recognizing the importance of nutrition. Most physicians at that time thought—if they thought about nutrition at all—that if you ate enough calories then you were well fed. McCollum recounts one dinner where he was asked to speak about nutrition. He spoke about his experiments with rats. After he sat down, an eminent physician said, slowly and clearly, "It doesn't matter what you eat. If you have long-lived ancestors you will have a long life."[7]

Despite the scorn of some physicians, this appointment was successful. Once at Johns Hopkins, McCollum continued his work with rats. His work led to the discovery of Vitamin D and will be discussed in that chapter. He carried photographs of his rats and showed them to anyone who was interested. His pictures of rats with eyes that were dry and inflamed because of Vitamin A deficiency attracted the most attention. In some ways this was misleading because the even greater importance of Vitamin A deficiency was its effect on the body's defenses against infection, which was not as visible as the red eyes of the rats.

McCollum developed another interest: educating the American public about a proper diet. In so doing, he departed from the usual role of the academic. Most scientists write articles for scientific or professional journals that concern technical points and can be difficult to read or to understand. Scientific articles are rarely "big picture" compositions. McCollum was convinced that his work with laboratory rats had important implications for the public. He became nutrition editor for *McCall's*, a monthly women's magazine, and wrote more than 160 articles for *McCall's*. (It is probable that some physicians were scornful of this also.)

McCollum also became a staunch opponent of fortification of food with vitamins. He was continuing in the steps of Stephen Babcock, who had never been comfortable with the Liebig idea that food was a mixture of laboratory chemicals. McCollum had begun his career by puzzling over the inability of scientists to predict the correct diet for cows. He respected the dairy farmers who insisted that their cows needed varied diets. He remembered this when switching to rodent and human diets. He advised the American housewife that varied diets containing many foods, especially dairy products, were the healthiest. He did not think that the American housewife should depend on chemicals to keep her family healthy.

Carotenoids and Vitamin A

McCollum and his group knew that green leafy vegetables also seemed to be rich in Vitamin A. This was not quite the case. In the 1930s, scientists showed that substances in plants, known as carotenoids, could be changed in the body to Vitamin A. β-Carotene, a bright-orange pigment, is the most common carotenoid with pro-Vitamin A activity. Green leafy vegetables also proved to be excellent sources of carotenoids.

CAROTENOIDS

Carotenoids are brightly colored pigments in plants, algae, and bacteria. They are usually yellow, orange, or red. Carotenoids are stable molecules that protect and assist chlorophyll in its role of photosynthesis. Photosynthesis is the means by which plants make sugar from water and carbon dioxide by using sunlight. Carotenoids are responsible for the bright colors of many vegetables and fruits and the vivid colors of autumn leaves.

There are at least six hundred types of carotenoids, about fifty of which can be changed to Vitamin A. β-Carotene is found in carrots, spinach, sweet potatoes, peaches, cantaloupes, and apricots. Without carotenoids, there would be no Vitamin A.

Formula and Synthesis of Vitamin A, Its Role in Vision, and Two Nobel Prizes

Paul Karrer (1889–1971) at the University of Zurich solved the chemical formula of β-carotene in 1930 and of Vitamin A in 1933. He was awarded the Nobel Prize in Chemistry in 1937 in recognition of this work. Vitamin A was synthesized in 1947. Beginning with McCollum, scientists had long noted the relationship between Vitamin A deficiency and eye problems.

George Wald (1906–1997), who had worked with Karrer, described Vitamin A in the retina of the frog and worked out the details of the cycle of pigment formation and breakdown in the eye. Vitamin A is needed for vision in dim light. In doing the work of "seeing" at night, the rods of the eye actually "use up" Vitamin A, so the diet must contain Vitamin A (see Appendix 1). He was awarded the Nobel Prize in Physiology, or Medicine, for this work in 1967.

Vitamin A and Anti-Infective Properties: Early Studies

McCollum had noted infections in rats not fed Vitamin A, as had other scientists, including Sir Edward Mellanby (1884–1955), a British physician and pharmacologist. Mellanby, who also worked with rickets, was so impressed with pneumonia in Vitamin A–deprived dogs that he called this vitamin the "anti-infective" vitamin. Were these findings relevant to humans? Three researchers from three countries in the early part of the twentieth century thought so, but then physicians forgot about this until the 1970s.

Masamichi Mori (1860–1932), a Japanese physician, graduated from the University of Tokyo School of Medicine and then studied in Germany and Switzerland from 1889 to 1905 before returning to Japan. In 1904 he described 1,511 cases of children with xerophthalmia, or "dry eye." These children lived in mountainous areas of Japan and ate mostly grains and vegetables. The children developed their eye problems after weaning. Later problems were diarrhea, weight loss, and dry skin. In more severe cases, the children had corneal ulcers and blindness. Mori noted that Japanese children rarely drank milk after weaning and that there were no fish in the mountains of Japan. The children recovered when given cod-liver oil, chicken liver, or eel fat.

Carl E. Bloch (1872–1952), a Danish pediatrician, made similar observations in Danish children, even though Denmark has many dairy cows. How could Danish children not consume enough Vitamin A? The answer had to do with wartime changes in food distribution. Butter was rare in Denmark during World War I because so much of it was exported. Margarine was used in its place. Bloch described forty cases of xerophthalmia in poorly fed children in Denmark between 1912 and 1916. They ate bread, potatoes, and centrifuged milk. The milk was centrifuged so that the fat rose to the top, and the butterfat was exported. The milk supplied to the children was fat free. Later, Bloch was responsible for thirty-two children in an orphanage. Only the children who received generous portions of butterfat thrived. The other children grew slowly and had many infections and eye problems. Bloch read McCollum's work and realized that he had encountered Vitamin A deficiency in children.

In London in the late 1920s and early 1930s, epidemics of measles were not uncommon. Children died from complications of measles, such as pneumonia and diarrhea. This may have been because the measles virus damages the epithelium throughout the body. (Epithelial cells form the outer layer of skin and the linings of eyes, lungs, and intestinal tracts. Intact linings serve as natural barriers against microorganisms.) When the measles virus damaged the epithelium, a common result was secondary infections causing pneumonia or diarrhea. These children who died from measles were often from destitute areas of London and were poorly fed.

J. B. Ellison, a young English physician, knew that work at Johns Hopkins showed that rats deprived of Vitamin A died of pneumonia. Ellison thought that the complications associated with measles were similar to those seen in the "devitaminized" rats. He organized a trial of six hundred children with measles, in which half of the children were treated with high doses of Vitamin A. These children were less likely to die from measles than the untreated children. This was one of the earliest controlled trials in medicine. It also highlighted the importance of Vitamin A in maintaining an intact epithelial barrier against infections.

Not all other researchers were able to find the same benefit from Vitamin A. There were other problems afflicting the same children who were Vitamin A deficient—poverty, poor sanitation, and inadequate immunization and vaccination programs—that made it difficult to focus on Vitamin A. The work of Mori, Bloch, and Ellison was not generally accepted and did not change medical thinking or practice.

Nutrition seemed to have little to do with infections and, with the development of antibiotics and vaccinations, interest in the connection between vitamins and infections became even weaker. Also, Vitamin A deficiency was unusual in wealthier countries. The finding that a lack of Vitamin A caused eye problems in rats and people was easier to grasp than was the idea that the vitamin could prevent infections. For some decades, the medical world was more interested in the effects of Vitamin A deficiency on vision than its effects on immunity.

Vitamin A and Anti-Infective Properties: Later Studies

Relatively recent work has been done with Vitamin A by another scientist from Johns Hopkins. Alfred Sommer (1942–) is an ophthalmologist who was studying night blindness and xerophthalmia in children in Indonesia between 1976 and 1980. He described an unexpected finding from the data:

> One December evening almost a year later, while a particular set of figures was being cross-tabulated, it became apparent that many xerophthalmic children were missing from later cross-tabulations. Running the computer analysis in the reverse direction revealed what the data had been waiting to tell us all along: children with even mild xerophthalmia were dying at a far greater rate.
>
> Any suggestion that the higher death rate was caused by malnutrition, of which the lack of Vitamin A was merely a symptom, was quickly dispelled. Malnutrition clearly increases the risk of child death, but so does Vitamin A deficiency—even among adequately nourished children. In fact the Indonesian study showed that malnourished children with adequate Vitamin A were less likely to die than well-nourished children who were deficient in Vitamin A.[8]

This finding was similar to what McCollum had found in his rats some decades earlier. Without Vitamin A, the rats did poorly and died. Sommer's figures confirmed Mori's findings in Japanese children and Bloch's findings in Danish orphans. Sommer and his team realized that night blindness was not a good marker of Vitamin A deficiency because it occurred only after the deficiency was severe. Even though Sommer, an ophthalmologist, had begun his work looking at eye diseases in children, he became interested in the unexpected deaths. He was walking down the same path traveled by his earlier Johns Hopkins colleague, Elmer McCollum.

Other researchers also found that children with Vitamin A eye problems were more likely to die from infections such as measles and diarrhea than were children without night blindness or xerophthalmia. Sommer and his team conducted large-scale epidemiological studies from 1983 to 1992, in which children received small doses of Vitamin A. Their vision improved, as did their general health. They developed measles and diarrhea just as often but were much less ill with these diseases.

In Africa, measles is a common and devastating childhood illness. Children who are Vitamin A deficient are more likely to become very ill with measles, and measles itself leads to Vitamin A deficiency. Sommer conducted a trial in hospitalized children with measles in Tanzania. Rates of deaths were lower in children with measles who were given large doses of Vitamin A by mouth. Similar studies were carried out by other researchers. This was a confirmation of Ellison's study four decades earlier.

Children in underdeveloped countries are those most likely to develop Vitamin A deficiency, which increases their susceptibility to infectious illnesses. The effects of the Vitamin A deficiency are often compounded by inadequate immunization programs and poor sanitation. Vitamin A deficiency occurs in more than two hundred fifty thousand children each year, resulting in blindness and a 50 percent mortality rate (primarily because of infectious illnesses) within the year. UNICEF now suggests that children with measles be treated with Vitamin A, and in 1993 the World Bank called the widespread use of Vitamin A one of the most cost-effective interventions in modern medicine.

SUMMARY

McCollum's decision to switch from cows to rats allowed him to distinguish between fats. He discovered that rats not fed with sufficient Vitamin A developed eye problems and infections. Other animal researchers confirmed these findings, and then Mori, Bloch, and Ellison made similar observations in children. Vitamin A's name, *retinol*, reflects the interest that scientists had in the vitamin's role in vision. The structure of the retina and its cones and rods and pigment cycles have captured the excitement of many scientists. The role of Vitamin A in maintaining our barriers against infections took a backseat to the eye interest for some years. This changed when a Johns

Hopkins ophthalmologist examined his cross-tabulations and rediscovered the anti-infective properties of this vitamin in work in Southeast Asia.

Vitamin A is needed for cell growth and division, particularly for the immune system, part of the body's system of defenses against bacteria and viruses, and for maintenance of the epithelial cells, natural barriers against microorganisms. Vitamin A supplementation is a cheap, easy, and important way of helping poorly fed children to survive infections, especially measles.

2

Soldiers in Pain and Staggering Chickens: Vitamin B1 (Thiamine), the Anti-Beriberi Vitamin

Overview

Thiamine was the first vitamin to be discovered. The story of thiamine is the story of beriberi, the disease caused by thiamine deficiency. Beriberi is associated with a diet consisting mainly of polished, or white, rice because the milling removes the thiamine. The disease occurs only in humans and in a small group of other animals, including chickens and pigeons. A major discovery was made thanks to the scruples of a cook who had strong beliefs about what was proper for chickens to eat. At least one of the beriberi researchers suffered pangs of conscience about the number of pigeons he sacrificed in the quest for the cure for beriberi. Many human prisoners were studied, and some also were experimented on, in the work to discover the cure for beriberi. Important work was done at the infamous Changi prisoner-of-war camp in Singapore during World War II.

Some people with beriberi can become quite confused and innocently make up stories. This is more likely to happen in people who are thiamine deficient and also alcoholic. Because people with alcoholism quite often eat poorly, thiamine deficiency may explain some of the brain damage associated with heavy and prolonged drinking of alcohol.

Beriberi

Beriberi is the illness that results from lack of thiamine. It is a complex illness that has two forms. In "wet" beriberi, the person suffers from heart problems and massive swelling of the legs. In "dry" beriberi, the person's legs are painful and weak, and walking is difficult. If the person is alcoholic or has lost weight quickly, dry beriberi also can be accompanied sometimes by confusion and memory loss. Both forms of the disease are associated with diets that consist mostly of rice.

Rice is an annual grass that grows in warm and wet areas. It is the dietary staple of much of the population in parts of Asia and Latin America, where labor and rain are plentiful. The rice seed is enclosed in an indigestible husk that must be removed before the rice can be eaten. Once the husk is removed, the grain is known as "brown rice" and is edible. Sometimes the brown skin, or pericarp, is removed to leave "white rice."

Different types of preparation of rice result in rice with varying amounts of thiamine:

- Removal of the husk by hand leads to brown rice with moderate thiamine.
- Removal of the husk and brown skin, or pericarp, by steel rollers leads to white rice with very little thiamine.
- Steaming, boiling, or soaking of the rice while it is still in the husk leads to parboiled rice with moderate thiamine.

The material removed from the rice is known as "rice polishings." Thiamine is contained in these polishings. The habit of washing rice vigorously sometimes results in the loss of thiamine as well.

Milling and Beriberi

Beriberi has existed for centuries in Southeast Asia among people whose diet was mainly rice. Until the 1800s rice was milled by hand to remove the indigestible husk. Hand milling was done on small quantities of rice on a daily basis. Not all of the skin or pericarp was removed, and the rice prepared this way had moderate amounts of thiamine.

In the nineteenth century, milling became mechanized. Around 1870 steel rollers for milling all types of grain were invented. Milling by machine was easier than milling by hand and removed one of the burdens of day-to-day life. Using these rollers, the outer layers of grain were removed much more thoroughly. This type of milling also removed more dirt, insects, and some of the grain fats, making the grain less likely to rot or become rancid during storage. The milled grains therefore had a longer "shelf life." People welcomed the freedom from daily milling and preferred the appearance, taste, and texture of milled grains. Machine-milled grain became associated with wealth and refinement.

This new technology was widely and quickly adopted but came with a price. More thiamine was removed from the rice with more thorough milling. As the technology spread, so did the illness beriberi. We shall see a similar sequence of events when we discuss pellagra.

The Dutch Colonies and Beriberi

Much of the Western knowledge of the illness comes from the work of Dutch physicians. The Netherlands was immensely wealthy in the seventeenth and eighteenth centuries, in large part because of its merchant marine. Amsterdam was the leading port in northern Europe. Dutch ships, sailors, and merchants traveled all over the globe and colonized parts of Southeast

Asia. The Dutch profited from the rich natural resources of these tropical regions.

One of the first Europeans to describe beriberi was a Dutch physician, Nicolaaes Tulp (1593–1674). He described the illness in a man who had been living in the Dutch East Indies. Jacobus Bontius (1592–1631), another Dutch physician, described cases of beriberi in Batavia, the capital of the Dutch East Indies, now known as Java. He himself developed the illness.

Beriberi in Japan

Beriberi, known as *kakké* ("leg disease" in Japanese), had existed in Japan for centuries. It became more common beginning in the 1700s, particularly in the Japanese navy. One third of enlisted men in the Japanese navy in the period between 1878 and 1882 were ill with beriberi. The Japanese assumed that bacteria caused the illness. They sent Kanehiro Takaki (1849–1920), a medical officer in the Japanese Imperial Navy, to St. Thomas' Medical Hospital in London, England, for further medical education that might help him to address the problem of beriberi. He mastered bacteriology, but he also learned about the health of the English navy. This turned out to be the more important part of his education. From Takaki's viewpoint, the English navy was remarkable in its freedom from beriberi. Takaki did not focus on bacteria. He thought that the relatively protein-rich diet protected the English navy from beriberi.

Takaki returned to Japan and tested his idea by changing the food supplied to the crew of a Japanese training ship. In 1882, this ship sailed from Japan to New Zealand and then along the western coast of South America to Honolulu. It returned to Japan in 1884. Takaki had convinced the authorities to supplement the crew's usual white rice–heavy diet with meat, milk, and vegetables. The change in diet was associated with a lower incidence of beriberi. He concluded that the low protein in the Japanese diets caused beriberi. The diet was changed throughout the Japanese navy, and the health of the Japanese seamen improved. Takaki was made a baron in recognition of this great achievement. However, his results had little influence on the rest of the world or even other branches of the Japanese military.

Physicians working in the Japanese army did not pay attention to the work of Takaki. The physicians working in the Japanese Army Medical Corps received their training at the University of Tokyo, which was allied with German medicine. German medicine, the best in the world at that time, was influenced by the work of Robert Koch (1843–1910), the physician who had discovered the bacteria that caused anthrax and tuberculosis. Japanese army physicians trained in Germany were not impressed by a navy physician trained in England. They did not believe that beriberi could be anything other than an infectious illness. Indeed, most physicians of the time thought that beriberi was infectious.

Investigations into Beriberi in the Dutch East Indies: Chickens with Spasms

The person associated with discovering the cause of beriberi is another Dutch physician. Christiaan Eijkman (1858–1930) studied at the Military Medical School of the University of Amsterdam, where he was trained as a medical officer for the Netherlands Indies Army. He received extra training in Berlin with Koch. Eijkman was sent out to Batavia to investigate the causes of beriberi. The Dutch colonial authorities in Indonesia were alarmed about the loss of so many of their soldiers to beriberi. Eijkman was not aware of Takaki's work and expected to discover the infectious cause of beriberi. He began his work with rabbits, injecting them with a micrococcus. The rabbits stayed well. Meanwhile, Eijkman noticed that chickens in his laboratory—in contrast to the healthy micrococcus-laden rabbits—were ill. The birds staggered and lost control of their wings. They had spasms in their muscles, which pulled their heads and necks backwards. Eijkman saw that this illness, which he named *polyneuritis gallinarum,* was similar to the polyneuritis occurring in people ill with beriberi. The encounter with beriberi in the staggering chickens was a stroke of good fortune. Beriberi does not occur in other animals often used in laboratories, such as dogs, rabbits, rats, or monkeys. Beriberi occurs only in humans, chickens, and pigeons. Eijkman had found one of the few animals that develops beriberi.

He examined and compared the peripheral nerves, the nerves that travel from the spinal cord to the rest of the body, from chickens with polyneuritis and humans ill with beriberi. In both chicken and human peripheral nerves, he saw a similar degeneration. His recognition of beriberi in chickens and then the confirmation of the similarity to human beriberi were brilliant achievements. Eijkman tried to capitalize on this finding by deliberately causing beriberi in his laboratory chickens. He inoculated them with material from patients ill with beriberi. His inoculated chickens did develop polyneuritis, but so did his uninoculated chickens. This was discouraging, but then the situation worsened. In 1889, just at the beginning of his investigations, beriberi in his chickens disappeared. Not only could he not cause the illness by transferring what should have been an infectious agent, but the chickens were no longer developing the illness. The chickens became well. Eijkman had found an animal model and then lost it.

Herein lay another example of Eijkman's brilliance. At this point, others would have cursed the chickens and their unreliable polyneuritis and given up. Eijkman saw the opportunity in this seeming disaster. Rather than being the end of his research, the disappearance of the polyneuritis was the clue to the illness. Eijkman discovered that a new cook had changed the diet fed to the chickens. The original chicken diet had come from the leftovers of the polished rice from the officers' table in the military hospital. This was rice that had been milled and, hence, more expensive and highly regarded than unmilled rice. The new cook had disapproved of the luxurious fowl diet. This cook believed that military rice should not be given to civilian chickens. The chicken diet returned to the lowly unpolished rice, and with this change, the chicken neuritis disappeared. This was a seemingly small change in their diet, and it is remarkable that this Dutch physician, who had trained with the world's leading medical researcher of the time and who was looking for an infectious agent, should have been interested in such mundane details as a chicken diet. It must have been difficult to think that the officers' diet was less healthy than the diet given to ordinary soldiers.

Eijkman had to be certain first of all that it really was the polished rice and not something else that he had overlooked. There were many possibilities:

• contaminated laboratory or cooking water;
• poison in the rice or a poisonous variety of rice;
• starvation; or
• insufficient fiber, protein, or salt in diet.

Eijkman tested and rejected all of these hypotheses. He concluded that the neuritis in chickens was indeed caused by polished, rather than unpolished, rice.

Why was the white rice so noxious to the chickens? Eijkman considered but rejected the idea of a nutritional deficiency in the white rice. He thought that the rice pericarp, which was lost in the milling process, contained some kind of antidote to poisons in the starch of the rice. He decided on another theory: that the rice pericarp provided a protective barrier to harmful microorganisms and that without this protection, the rice grain was contaminated. Therefore, as we now know, he did not quite realize what he had discovered. He had the answer in his hands, and it fell through his fingers. Nonetheless, his use of chicken polyneuritis as a way of investigating beriberi and his observation of the importance of a change in type of rice that was fed to chickens changed the way that people understood this illness.

Eijkman Struggles with Dutch Chickens and Angry Colleagues

Eijkman returned to the Netherlands in 1896 because he was ill with malaria. Once home, his health improved, but his scientific life deteriorated. He was unable to replicate his Indonesian findings with Dutch chickens. He imported chickens from Indonesia—still no luck. Finally, he discovered that the chickens in Holland—whether Dutch or Indonesian—did not like to eat white rice. Eijkman changed his tactics. He forced the white rice down their crops and they developed the neuritis. The chickens were not making his life easy, nor were his colleagues. They were outraged at his dismissal of their beriberi theories and responded with personal attacks. Eijkman recorded one comment: "If one considers that Eijkman apparently needed six years in order to do this work, it must be considered the most inadequate product which can be found in the literature from the Director of a scientific institute."[1]

Eijkman pointed out to some of his critics that they had not been to Southeast Asia and so perhaps did not know as much about beriberi as he did, to which his critics replied that "the opinions of 'colonials' could not be given much weight, since they had all been eating rice and their brains were therefore damaged."[2] Eijkman, no doubt tiring of force-feeding his chickens while being insulted by his colleagues, declared that beriberi was an infectious illness and retired from the battle. He devoted the remainder of his career to other matters. Although Eijkman drew the wrong conclusions, his work, unlike that of Takaki, did have a great impact on other scientists. He was awarded the 1929 Nobel Prize in Medicine, or Physiology, in recognition of his work.

Vorderman and Grijns Continue Eijkman's Work

Eijkman had discussed his findings with A. G. Vorderman, a physician who was inspector of prisons in Java. In the late 1800s, Java was one of the most densely populated areas in the world. The population was between thirty and thirty-five million, and almost 1 percent of the population was in prison. Vorderman was intrigued by his friend's findings and realized that there was a natural experiment taking place in his 101 prisons. It was already known that beriberi was a problem in some but not all prisons. Vorderman and Eijkman had the opportunity to see if what was true for Eijkman's chickens was true for Java's prisoners. In prisons, the supply of food was controlled. It was fairly easy to determine what the prisoners were eating and to identify which prisoners became ill with beriberi. Vorderman surveyed the diets of nearly 280,000 prisoners in all of the 101 prisons in 1896. The result was clear: beriberi was most common in the prisons that gave their prisoners a diet consisting mostly of polished rice. Vorderman agreed with Eijkman that beriberi was an infectious disease and that the problem with the white rice diet was that it decreased resistance to the infectious agent, whatever that agent was.

Meanwhile, another Dutch military doctor, Gerrit Grijns (1885–1944), took Eijkman's place in Batavia. Grijns continued Eijkman's work, but from a different angle. Perhaps having the advantage of a fresh perspective, Grijns saw beriberi not as an illness because of toxins in the rice but as a deficiency disease. Grijns worked with nearly 250 birds for five years. In his publications, one can follow each bird's fate, bird by bird. He found that supplementing the chickens' diet with peas was effective in treating chicken beriberi. He was one of the first to understand that a disease could result from the deficiency of a factor that was, at the time, too small to identify or to measure and that could not be replaced by known chemical compounds. This was difficult to comprehend at the time.

British Investigators Conduct Experiments in Malaya, and Some Attendees at an International Conference Blame Beriberi on Rice

British investigators became interested because beriberi was problematic in Malaya, then a British-controlled territory. They carried out a number of studies that confirmed the observations of Vorderman. In 1905, William

Fletcher (1874–1938), a British bacteriologist who had trained at Cambridge, examined beriberi in an experiment in a psychiatric hospital in Kuala Lampur, Malaya. Psychiatric hospitals in those days were large institutions somewhat like prisons, in that the patients stayed for months or years, and the experimenter could be fairly sure about their diet. Beriberi was a problem in this hospital. Fletcher organized a trial to try to *disprove* the suggestion that parboiled rice was superior to white rice. One ward was supplied with white rice, and one was supplied with parboiled rice. Beriberi was more common in the white rice ward. Fletcher changed his mind and decided that beriberi was *not* infectious. He was unsure as to what the exact cause of beriberi could be.

Henry Fraser, a Scottish physician, and Thomas Stanton, a Canadian physician, carried out a clever experiment in a different population in 1907. They studied Javanese road builders in two camps in remote areas of Malaya. The laborers were healthy and lived in camps far from other populations. The laborers were unlikely to be infected by any organisms that might cause beriberi. Until their work was finished, the laborers could not easily leave the work camps. Fraser and Stanton informed the men that parboiled rice was suspected to be healthier than white rice. The laborers preferred the white rice. They were good subjects—healthy, isolated, informed, and trapped. One half of the men were given white rice, the better tasting diet, and one half were given parboiled rice, the rice thought to be healthier. This study seems less exploitative than the work with the mentally ill, in that the laborers were warned of the dangers of white rice. Fraser and Stanton found that laborers fed parboiled rice were indeed less likely to develop beriberi. In separate experiments, they also found that alcohol extracts of parboiled rice cured the illness in chickens fed with white rice. Fraser and Stanton suggested, along the same lines as Grijns, that the polished white rice lacked "some substance or substances essential for the normal metabolism of nerve tissues."

There was now international interest in tropical illnesses in Southeast Asia. The Far Eastern Association of Tropical Medicine was held in Manila in March 1910. Beriberi was the first item on the agenda. National pride became involved. Japan took exception to the general finger-pointing at rice. Takaki had made great progress in showing that beriberi was associated with nutrition but never "blamed" the illness on white rice. He thought that low protein was the problem. However, by the end of the meeting, the Association did conclude that beriberi was connected with white rice. It is thought that Japan left the conference early. This is a lesson not to leave meetings prematurely.

American Investigators and a Disastrous Experiment with Bubonic Plague: For Their Next Experiment, They Get Written Consent

Americans now became drawn into beriberi research because of their colonization of the Philippines. Richard Pearson Strong (1872–1948) organized a nutritional trial involving prisoners in the Bilibid prison in Manila. This experiment was one of the first to involve written and signed consent. The background for this was an unexpected outbreak of the bubonic plague. Strong, an American physician, had graduated from the first medical class at Johns Hopkins in 1897. He had later studied in Germany and then went to Southeast Asia, where he became director of the Biological Laboratory of the Philippine Bureau of Science. Before his work with beriberi, he had been interested in devising a cholera vaccine. In 1906, he inoculated twenty-four Bilibid prisoners with cholera vaccine. The point of the inoculation was to assess the side effects associated with this particular vaccine and not, in fact, to protect them from cholera. No one explained to the prisoners the purpose of the experiment or asked their permission. All of the prisoners were Filipino. Ten of twenty-four prisoners died from bubonic plague. An investigation revealed that test tubes with active bubonic plague had been mixed up with tubes containing cholera vaccine. The cholera vaccine and active plague tubes had been stored in the same incubator. Perhaps this played a part in the blunder. Strong blamed a visiting Dutch physician. Japanese carpenters who had been working in the area were also suspected. The thinking was clear: anonymous foreigners, rather than Americans, must have been responsible. There was an outcry among some Americans, particularly those already apprehensive about America becoming a colonial power and sensitive to the possibility of Filipinos being treated badly.

Strong continued his work with Bilibid prisoners but never worked with cholera vaccine or bubonic plague again. He also changed some of his methods. He began to do nutritional experiments with the prisoners to see whether he could advance the field of beriberi research. He decided to compare the effects of feeding prisoners a diet of white rice with or without rice polishings. Twenty-nine men, all sentenced to death, "agreed" to participate in his new study. The prisoners who participated in this trial signed documents that explained the experiment and the voluntary nature of it. The documents were written in their dialects. In return for their participation, they were offered cigarettes and cigars. (This illustrates the strong appeal of nicotine.) For about three months, one group was fed mostly polished white rice. The other group was fed white rice with either rice polishings, which turned out to be inedible, or white rice with the addition of an alcoholic extraction of rice polishings. One man died. His autopsy showed acute beriberi. He had been in the group fed polished white rice. Eight men in the polished white rice group developed beriberi, but no one in the other two groups became ill. This was a landmark study because the prisoners gave written consent. The study showed once again that the illness was related to polished rice, but this theory still was not generally accepted because of the great appeal of the theory that bacteria caused illnesses.

Laboratory Work in England and Argument about a Word

Hopkins had demonstrated the existence of "accessory factors" that were important for nutrition and had lectured about them in 1912, as was reviewed in the Vitamin A chapter, but he did not use the word "vitamin." The Polish–American biochemist Casimir Funk (1884–1967) was responsible for this word. Funk had trained in Europe and then moved to England, where he worked at the Lister Institute in London on the beriberi problem. He thought that he had identified the anti-beriberi substance in unpolished rice as an amine (see glossary) and named it "vitamine," i.e., "vital amine," in 1912. (He had actually identified what would later be known as niacin.) He then boldly suggested that "vitamine" be used as the word for all of the mysterious food factors that were related to deficiency diseases. He was sure that all of these factors would turn out to be amines.

The new word became popular, but not with other nutritional experts such as McCollum and Hopkins. Infighting between the rivals occurred. Funk claimed that only substances that cured beriberi and scurvy deserved the name "vitamine." McCollum insisted that only his fat-soluble growth factor (later to be named Vitamin A) and what would later be called thiamine were vitamins. Only Funk was certain that these substances or factors would all be amines. Eventually, as we will see in the Vitamin C chapter, the new word "vitamin" was proposed. This spelling change was accepted by everyone, with the exception of Funk, who continued to use his word "vitamine."

Although Funk was wrong about the anti-beriberi substance, he was correct in understanding that unpolished rice contained a vital substance. He also accurately predicted that pellagra—then a mysterious disease—would prove to be a deficiency disease. Funk was a creative and enthusiastic scientist who campaigned vigorously to get his word and idea accepted. Eventually, all agreed that there were multiple vitamins. This laboratory work and the new word were helpful in allowing scientists to understand the problem of beriberi. Hopkins, McCollum, and Funk had each formulated a theoretical framework for the connection between nutrition and disease that was compelling and, importantly, allowed for much future experimentation. Vanishingly small substances were important for health, just as were the more easily understood protein, carbohydrates, and fats.

Second Meeting of the Far Eastern Association of Tropical Medicine and the Search for the Molecule

The second meeting of the Far Eastern Association of Tropical Medicine took place in 1912 in Hong Kong. Once again, beriberi was the main topic. Many still believed that the illness was infectious, but all present agreed that white polished rice was associated with the illness and that addition of rice bran or consumption of less milled rice prevented the illness. The question that faced the experts was simple: What was the substance in the rice skin or pericarp that was removed by milling that led people to develop beriberi? Two Dutchmen, B. C. P. Jansen and W. F. Donath, working in the Eijkman Institute in Batavia, Java, worked out a laborious procedure:

> After the initial extraction of 300 kg (or roughly 660 lb) of rice polishings with water, the active factor was first absorbed from the extract onto a special kind of clay, then washed out with barium hydroxide and successively precipitated

with silver nitrate, phosphotungestic acid, platinic chloride, acetone, and picrolonic acid. After each precipitation and filtration, the factor had to be redissolved, in most cases with barium hydroxide. Finally, 100 mg of crystals were obtained with hydrochloric acid. From comparative bioassays of the crystals and starting material, it appeared that over 90 percent of the vitamin originally present had been lost during the process. Even Jansen and Donath had difficulties in obtaining crystals in subsequent runs.[3]

In summary, Jansen and Donath found 100 mg of thiamine in 300 kg of rice polishings in 1926. The process was temperamental and unreliable. Even after all this work, they were not able to determine the chemical structure of thiamine. (They did not realize that it contained a sulfur atom.)

Beriberi in Newfoundland and More Disagreements

An epidemic of beriberi broke out in Newfoundland, Canada, a part of the world remote in most ways from Southeast Asia. An Irish physician described the outbreak. Wallace Ruddell Aykroyd (1899–1979) trained in medicine in Ireland and in 1924 moved to Newfoundland. The Newfoundlanders were an ideal population to study. They fished, but they sold their fish abroad and ate little of it themselves. The rocky soil of Newfoundland grew little, and the island was snow-or ice-bound and inaccessible for six months of the year. As a result, the Newfoundlanders imported food, and Aykroyd easily established the content of their diet. It was almost as though they were living in an institution with a regulated food supply. Aykroyd discovered that beriberi struck in fishing communities in spring as the winter's food supply was becoming exhausted. Poor families depending on white bread, salt meat, and molasses were most likely to become ill.

Aykroyd saw beriberi as a problem of poverty. He had little patience for those who investigated the details of preparation of rice. Perhaps this was because, unusually in the history of beriberi, rice was not connected with the illness in Newfoundland. He noted, sharply, that administrators should pay more attention to poverty rather than the details of rice preparation.[4] However, in later years, Aykroyd joined company with people he had formerly disparaged. He fell prey to the seductive powers of the question of how to prepare rice. Despite his background in Newfoundland, he too published articles about the effects of parboiling and milling on the nutritional qualities of rice.[5]

Williams Discovers the Structure of Thiamine, Worries about the Pigeons, and Synthesizes the Vitamin

An American physician, Edward Bright Vedder (1878–1952) of the U.S. Army Medical Corps in the Philippines, was aware of Grijns' and Eijkman's work. He also heard Fraser and Stanton present their findings at the 1910 Manila meeting. Vedder treated beriberi in babies successfully with rice polishings. He became determined to find out what it was in the rice polishings that treated beriberi. Vedder recruited a young chemist, Robert Runnels Williams (1886–1965), to help him in this project. Williams was a peripatetic man of eclectic interests and diverse abilities. He was born in India to American missionaries and received graduate training in chemistry at the University of Chicago. He later went to the Philippines, where he met Vedder, who introduced him to the problem of beriberi. Williams worked at the Bureau of Science in Manila in attempts to find the beriberi-preventing substance but did not succeed. He left the Philippines in 1915 and joined what is now known as the Food and Drug Administration of the U.S. government. During World War I, he worked in chemical warfare and later in research problems in the Air Service. In 1919, Williams left the government and worked on submarine cable insulation for Bell Laboratory. It must have seemed that he had abandoned the problem assigned to him by Vedder.

However, the Great Depression of the 1930s allowed him to return to his earlier project. During the Depression, Bell Labs could not afford to employ Williams full time. He used this opportunity to pursue his true interest. He worked part time for Bell, and during his extra time, he returned to the problem of beriberi. He kept pigeons in the garage in his own home. He obtained small grants from the Fleischmann Company and then Carnegie. He set up a copper-screened rotor in his family washing machine and turned it into a dialysis machine. The work was difficult for several reasons. Williams had to be careful that his various experimental diets caused pure beriberi rather than another nutritional disease. The diet had to lack the antineuritic vitamin, but no other. The laboratory animals did not always become ill in ways that were helpful to the work at hand. Williams describes this problem:

> In later years I worked with a total of well over a thousand pigeons and came more and more to mistrust any single curative experiment with them. They do indeed succumb to polyneuritis rather more rapidly than chickens, that is, in as little as fourteen days. The symptoms in pigeons are also highly dramatic. The neck contortions and their violent and uncontrollable floppings when prodded into action during a polyneuritic crisis are indeed unmistakable signs. However, as my experience extended to larger numbers I frequently saw pigeons go through violent contortions of this sort at one hour of the day but spontaneously recover temporarily a few hours later. This improvement might well last in some cases for one to three days; but, more often, the bird would be dead the following morning.
>
> Pigeons, also, vary greatly in the rapidity with which they develop forthright symptoms and in respect to the character of their symptoms. I have sometimes had batches of a dozen pigeons, every one of which developed striking symptoms within four weeks. In other equal lots from the same source half or even nearly all of them would merely gradually grow thinner and weaker and be found dead without ever having shown an unmistakable symptom . . . I am far from confident that the God of pigeons will forgive me in the next world for all the hundreds or thousands of pigeons I futilely slaughtered during the twelve years I relied upon them as test animals.[6]

This is somewhat similar to the situation with Eijkman's Dutch chickens. Experimental animals rarely behave as well as the researcher believes that they should.

Williams was carried away by unreasonable self-doubt and self-recrimination when he wrote the above passage. His work was not futile. The deaths of the pigeons were not in vain (at least not from the human point of view). Despite the unpredictable and histrionic behavior on the part of the pigeons, Williams succeeded in 1933 in determining the structure of thiamine, ahead of his many competitors. A short three years later, he had synthesized thiamine. Williams patented each and every step in his work and used the royalties to support further research. In 1938, he wrote *Vitamin B1 and Its Use in Medicine* with a colleague, Thomas Spies.

Beriberi in World War II, Common in Prisoner-of-War Camps, Disappears from Newfoundland

Beriberi remained a serious and common illness in the Far East. It was the main cause of death among American and British prisoners of war in Japanese camps during World War II in the Philippines and Burma, where the diet consisted mainly of rice. At least one of the prisoners of war understood the illness, thanks to Williams and Spies. Singapore fell to the Japanese in February 1942, and over fifty thousand Allied troops were prisoners of war at the Changi camp in Singapore for three and a half years. The experience of these troops is the basis of the novel *King Rat* by James Clavell (himself a prisoner in the camp.) Clavell describes the monotonous rice-based diet, the constant hunger the men faced, their fear of beriberi, and the various Machiavellian tricks practiced by some of the prisoners to obtain more and better quality food. Had he wanted to describe man at his best, rather than at his worst, he could have described different activities. (Perhaps he would not then have had a best seller.) He could have described a bibliographic and nutritional feat of bravery.

Some of the prisoners at Changi were doctors who were aware of the recent findings of Williams and others. For example, R. C. Burgess was a prisoner of war at Changi for three and a half years and saw the illness begin in many of his coprisoners. He managed to get a message to a Chinese sympathizer who smuggled Williams' book, *Vitamin B1 and Its Use in Medicine*, into the camp. Burgess read the book and as a result changed the way rice was prepared. He discouraged the overly vigorous washing of the polished rice. Any water that was used to wash the rice was reused for soup. Thus, by drinking the thiamine-containing wash water, the prisoners were able to get some thiamine. Burgess saved thousands of lives in this way. Burgess and others wrote scientific articles about the effects of vitamin deprivation on the health of the prisoners. They were able to estimate the nutritional content of the food and perform meticulous physical examinations.[7]

Meanwhile, World War II was good for the health of the Newfound-landers. Beriberi disappeared from Newfoundland because World War II led to the expansion of the airport at Gander, which was necessary for planes making the long transatlantic trip. This led to greater employment, which in turn led to higher standards of living and better and more variety of food. The thiamine levels of the Newfoundlanders rose, and beriberi disappeared.

Thiamine Fortification of Foods: Improving Our Ability to Kill Others

Thiamine has been added to grain products in the United States and most other countries in the developed world for the last several decades. This is partly because of concern about the health of soldiers and the civilian popula-tion in World War II. In May 1941, President Roosevelt arranged a National Nutrition Conference for Defense. This was prompted by the dismaying find-ings of ill health among young men who were enlisting for military service. About one quarter of these men were found to be unfit because of malnutri-tion. An equal if not greater number of babies, younger children, women, and elderly were almost certainly also malnourished. At that time, many grains were thoroughly milled. The Conference recommended that low-cost staples such as flour and bread be refortified with the "lost nutritive ele-ments." The goal was to ensure that all Americans, no matter what their income, would eat enough food with vitamins. On January 1, 1942, the Food and Drug Administration recommended that white flour be fortified with iron, thiamine, and niacin. Over the next few years, pasta, white bread, corn-meal, grits, and white rice were enriched also with iron, riboflavin, niacin, and thiamine. These changes were mandated during the war and afterwards left to the discretion of the individual states. It is difficult to escape the irony of this. The government became alarmed at widespread malnutrition among young men, fearing that they would not be fit enough to wound, maim, or kill other young men. Americans have become much healthier since then. Per-haps this is due to the generally improved diet and greater attention to vari-ety of foods and refrigeration. Has food fortification been necessary? An international unintended experiment answered this question in part.

Beriberi, Alcoholism, and Australia

Bread was not fortified with thiamine in Australia as early as it was in other countries. An expert committee in that country had concluded that the aver-age Australian diet contained enough thiamine. They did recognize that Aus-tralian alcoholics were not consuming enough thiamine. The committee wrote in 1959 that "it would be wrong in principle to add a substance to bread in order to treat a minority which is suffering from a disease—alcoholism. Better methods for treating this problem should be sought."[8] This principled approach provided nutritionists and clinicians with a geographic natural experiment. Autopsies done in the 1980s showed that the prevalence of thiamine deficiency syndromes such as Wernicke-Korsakoff syndrome (discussed below) was much higher in Australia than in other countries that enriched their bread. Despite the recommendations of the committee, "better methods for treating this problem" were never found. Policy was reversed, and Australian millers added thiamine to their products. Once bread was fortified in Australia, in 1991, the incidence of thiamine-related disorders decreased to levels seen in other developed countries.[9] The Australians deserted their principles, and their alcoholics became healthier.

Should Rice Be Enriched?

R. R. Williams combined great research ability with a drive to see laboratory advances translated into practice. He organized a large-scale trial of rice enrichment in Bataan in the Philippines in 1948. Surprisingly, this was controversial. Nutritional experts at the United Nations believed that a more appropriate approach was to improve nutritional status by increasing the diversity of foods. They also argued that greater attention should be paid to the socioeconomic circumstances of the population. Some experts claimed that the Bataan trial had failed, and others argued that it had succeeded. Williams' patents raised suspicions. Half a century later, it seems obvious that both sides were correct. At the time, however, there was much bitterness.

Beriberi and the Brain

Wernicke-Korsakoff syndrome is a thiamine deficiency syndrome that is usually described in alcoholics. Something in the interaction between alcohol and a thiamine deficiency is uniquely toxic to the brain.

Wernicke and His Triad

Carl Wernicke (1848–1905) was a Polish-born neurologist who studied and worked in Germany. In 1881, he described a constellation of symptoms in three people: two alcoholic men and a young seamstress who had swallowed sulfuric acid in a suicide attempt and then had persistent vomiting. They experienced three characteristic symptoms—ataxia, confusion, and opthalmoplegia—a weakness of the eye muscles. This became known as Wernicke's encephalopathy, or brain disorder. All died within a few weeks. Wernicke's triad has become well known in medical textbooks:

1. Ataxia: inability to walk smoothly or maintain balance;
2. Confusion: difficulty in thinking clearly; and
3. Opthalmoplegia: jerky eye movements or difficulty in moving eyes from side to side.

Korsakoff and Making up Stories

Eight years later, in 1889, Sergei Sergeievich Korsakoff (1853–1900), a Russian psychiatrist working in Moscow, described a peculiar form of amnesia, often associated with a wide variety of psychiatric symptoms, in twenty alcoholic patients who also suffered from damage to their peripheral nerves. He suggested that one mechanism damaged both the peripheral nerves and the brain. He also described the syndrome of loss of short-term memory and confabulation in a classic work published the same year. Korsakoff was the first person to describe this syndrome. Confabulation is the name for the disorder in which the person makes up stories. The person who confabulates is unaware that he or she is doing so. Imagination is mistaken for memory. Confabulation is different from lying, because the person believes what he or she is saying and does not profit from the untruth. Confabulation is also different from psychosis in that the stories are not particularly bizarre, and the person does not hear voices or see things that others do not. Korsakoff described a syndrome that he had seen in several patients with chronic alcoholism or severe vomiting:

> At first, during conversation with such a patient, it is difficult to note the presence of psychic disorder; the patient gives the impression of a person in complete possession of his faculties; he reasons about everything perfectly well, draws correct deductions from given premises, makes witty remarks, plays chess or a game of cards, in a word, comports himself as a mentally sound person. Only after a long conversation with the patient, one may note that at times he utterly confuses events and that he remembers absolutely nothing of what goes on around him: he does not remember whether he had his dinner, whether he was out of bed. On occasion the patient forgets what happened to him just an instant ago: you came in, conversed with him, and stepped out for one minute; then you come in again and the patient has absolutely no recollection that you had already been with him. Patients of this type may read the same page over and again sometimes for hours, because they are absolutely unable to remember what they have read . . . the patients usually remember quite accurately the past events which occurred long before the illness . . . he would tell that yesterday he took a ride in town, whereas in fact he has been in bed for two months, or he would tell of conversations which have never occurred. . . .[10]

This became known as Korsakoff's psychosis. This is a misleading name because there is no psychosis in Korsakoff's psychosis. There are no hallucinations or delusions. The main problem in this disorder is that the person cannot form new memories. As noted by Korsakoff, the person may be able to play chess or a game of cards but would not be able to say with any accuracy when their last meal was. Once Korsakoff's psychosis has developed, the person is unable to live independently.

Conjunction of the Two Disorders

The recognition of the full Wernicke-Korsakoff syndrome was difficult, in part because it is usually found in alcoholics with many nutritional deficiencies and other alcohol-caused problems or in very ill people with a multitude of medical problems. Over time, physicians came to realize that if Wernicke's encephalopathy is not treated, the person develops Korsakoff's psychosis. As we now know, different aspects of one syndrome had been described by these two men. In a rare spirit of international goodwill, it came to be known as the Wernicke-Korsakoff syndrome. Wernicke-Korsakoff syndrome today is usually seen in people with alcoholism, particularly men. It is often not diagnosed because of the person's intoxication. Alcoholic men have many reasons to eat poorly:

- Loss of appetite because alcohol is dense in calories;
- Poverty because of inability to keep job;
- Isolation because of inability to maintain relationships;
- Depression, which itself interferes with appetite, work, and relationships.

Although usually found in alcoholics, the Wernicke-Korsakoff syndrome occurs in other conditions associated with an inadequate diet. The syndrome has been described in prisoners of war. Eric Cruickshank, another researcher-physician-prisoner at the Changi camp, recorded details of about four hundred cases of beriberi. Eleven of the twelve men who developed Wernicke-Korsakoff syndrome were alcoholics. It has also been seen in people on fad diets or in anyone with poor nutrition.

Beriberi and Persistent Vomiting: The Woman Who Described a Meal of Steak and Potatoes, Salad with Blue Cheese Dressing, and Chocolate Cream Pie

As noted above, one of the first patients diagnosed with Wernicke's encephalopathy was a young woman who had swallowed sulfuric acid and then developed persistent vomiting. Any condition associated with persistent vomiting can lead to Wernicke-Korsakoff syndrome. Nutritional problems related to vitamin deficiencies in the past were usually because of inadequate amounts or variety of food, but in the developed world, obesity is now the major nutritional problem. Dieting and exercise are difficult. Surgical approaches to treat obesity are now used. Occasionally, vitamin deficiency can result from these more aggressive approaches.

Two common types of weight loss surgery are gastric bypass and adjustable gastric banding. Gastric bypass is a permanent rerouting of the digestive system. The stomach becomes a small pouch, and food bypasses the upper twenty to sixty inches of the small intestine. In adjustable gastric banding, the stomach is "banded" to form a small pouch with a restricted opening to the rest of the stomach. After these operations, it is uncomfortable to eat large amounts of food because of the smaller size of the stomach. Loss of part of the small intestine means that there is less bowel where food can be absorbed. The person both *eats* and *absorbs* less food. The reduction in food intake, frequent vomiting, and loss of absorptive surface after obesity-reducing surgery puts these patients at risk for multiple vitamin deficiencies. Thiamine deficiency, because it can result in permanent brain damage, is the most serious. Wernicke-Korsakoff syndrome is missed in alcoholics and is sometimes not diagnosed in people after weight loss surgery. Wernicke's triad, like all triads, has great teaching appeal and is beloved of medical students and their teachers. When it comes to clinical practice, however, the triad is often forgotten and the diagnosis made too late.

Harold Klawans, a neurologist, described a case of a thirty-two-year-old woman, Pat, who was very overweight and had had weight loss surgery. After the surgery, she developed persistent vomiting. Pat's vomiting was so severe that she stopped eating altogether. She lost over 130 pounds and developed burning feet. She was unable to walk smoothly. Several doctors saw her. Klawans describes a meeting Pat had with her surgeon and then a consulting neurologist:

> Pat did not recognize [her surgeon]. In fact, she had no idea where she was. She told him she hadn't vomited in weeks. And she told him all about the wonderful meal she'd eaten the night before, describing it in detail: steak and potatoes, salad with blue cheese dressing, and chocolate cream pie . . . She thought she was in a hotel. A man named Red Faber was with her. [Her neurologist] asked her if she was still vomiting. Of course not. Had she had lunch? Yes. What? Meat loaf, gravy, mashed potatoes, salad, cake, and two rolls with butter . . . In his note, [the neurologist] remarked that her excellent dietary history made any vitamin deficiency unlikely. Especially since her feet were no longer bothering her . . .
>   [Her malpractice lawyer described her condition a few days later.]
>   . . . She could not walk without assistance. She could talk but she couldn't remember much of anything that was new. She remembered almost everything up to about the time of her surgery. Since then, nothing.[11]

Doctors who read this anecdote will pay particular attention to the presence of the malpractice lawyer.

Pat's burning feet were part of dry beriberi. As her illness progressed, she became confused. She had ataxia and jerky eye movements. She had all three elements of the triad. Because she was not treated in time, the full Wernicke-Korsakoff syndrome developed. She began to confabulate about meals she had eaten and people that she had met. She forgot that her feet hurt. Her confusion confused her doctors, who believed that she had been eating properly. Therefore, they did not think that she needed thiamine, and her brain damage increased. She spent the rest of her life in an institution. This is the consequence of thiamine deficiency.

Summary

In the late 1800s, Eijkman and Grijns in the Dutch East Indies discovered that the cause of beriberi was a diet that relied too heavily on white rice, particularly if it had been mechanically milled. Williams did much laboratory work, thanks in part to the Great Depression, and worked out the formula of thiamine and fortified rice in the Philippines. Wernicke, Korsakoff, and physician-prisoners in the Changi prisoner-of-war camp described the clinical symptoms of thiamine deficiency. Thiamine deficiency combined with rapid weight loss and/or alcoholism can lead to confusion and memory loss. Thiamine deficiency is most common now in the setting of chronic alcoholism or in acute starvation syndromes.

3

DERMATITIS, DIARRHEA, DEMENTIA, AND DEATH: VITAMIN B3, (NIACIN), THE ANTI-PELLAGRA VITAMIN

OVERVIEW

The discovery of niacin, or Vitamin B3, was a result of the introduction of American maize, or corn, to the Western world. When diets consist mostly of corn, a vitamin deficiency illness, pellagra, can result. Pellagra was one of the unappreciated consequences of the European conquest of the Americas and became common in poor communities in Italy, France, Spain, and Egypt for nearly two centuries. In the United States, it was widespread among inmates of asylums and cotton-mill workers in the South. In 1937, the anti-pellagra vitamin was identified as nicotinic acid, a chemical which had been used in photography for several decades. The name was changed to *niacin* when bread was fortified with the vitamin so that people would not think that bread had been fortified with nicotine.

Interest surged in niacin in the early 1950s from an unexpected group of people—psychiatrists in the Canadian prairies. Researchers in Saskatoon, Saskatchewan, reported good results in treatment of schizophrenia with high doses of niacin. They also discovered that high doses of niacin lower cholesterol. Physicians today are more likely to use niacin to lower cholesterol than to treat schizophrenia. Niacin is different from the other vitamins in that humans can make it from tryptophan, an essential amino acid. This complicated the research—tryptophan-rich diets cured pellagra, but so did yeast, which contains no tryptophan at all. Most people need to consume niacin to have enough of this vitamin.

MAIZE

Maize in Central and South America

Maize, or corn, is a tall grass (*Zea mays*) originating in the highlands of central Mexico many thousands of years ago. Corn is now the dominant agricultural product of the United States and supports much of the American economy. Maize was the basic food plant of the Mayas, Aztecs, and Incas, who developed sophisticated civilizations in Central and South America. The Mayan people had a written language, understood the concepts of the calendar and zero, and built canals and irrigation systems. The Aztecs built beautiful cities with markets and canals. The Incas created monuments and intricate communication systems. All of these peoples had complex religious rituals and rich artistic cultures. The high caloric yield of the corn plant allowed these civilizations to flourish.

Corn and Photosynthesis

One of the reasons for the success of corn is its unusual photosynthetic pathway. In the 1970s, the world of photosynthesis research was rocked by an unexpected discovery. Scientists learned that corn actually has a different method of photosynthesis than other plants do. Corn produces more organic matter than do other plant species because of its more efficient method of photosynthesis.

These civilizations have all collapsed. The Mayan empire disappeared for unclear reasons, and the Aztecs and Incas were conquered by the Spanish. The Spanish conquest led to many changes in both the Americas and Europe. The Spanish conquistadors came to Central and South America in the fifteenth and sixteenth centuries looking for gold. The Native Americans valued gold for its use in jewelry and other artistic and religious objects. The conquistadors lusted for gold in ways that must have seemed very odd to the Native Americans—they wanted gold for itself.

Hernán Cortés (1485–1547) conquered Montezuma and the Aztecs, and his contemporary Francisco Pizarro (ca. 1471–1541) defeated the Incas. In both cases, the Spanish conquistadors were vastly outnumbered by the armies they were attacking but had other advantages. The conquistadors had horses and superior weapons—guns and swords made of steel. They also carried germs unfamiliar to the Aztecs and Incas. The Aztecs and Incas had no defenses against the horses, weapons, or germs.

The real treasure that the victorious Spaniards took back from Mexico and Peru was not the gold ingots fashioned from the Aztec and Incan religious objects, or even the few stolen artifacts. The real treasure of the Aztecs and Incas was another yellow object—corn. The transfer of maize from America to Europe does not have the same human drama as do the various battles and stories of treachery and bravery, but it is more important. Corn was both a blessing and a curse to the Spanish. Corn has been described as the "New World's single most important contribution to the human diet,"[1] yet as a gift, it was a Trojan Horse. It brought calories to the Old World, but they were calories unaccompanied by vitamins. Native Americans knew how to use maize wisely, but this knowledge did not accompany the corn to the New World.

Maize in North America: "The Three Sisters"

When the English pilgrims came to North America, they, like the conquistadors, found a populated land. The Indian tribes in the Northeast had created a democratic government in which women had an equal voice with men. Corn was the main crop for these communities in the eastern parts of North America. Corn was usually grown along with beans and squash. This system of agriculture was known as the "three sisters." Soil was mounded, corn was planted in the center of this mound, and then beans and squash were planted around the edges. The vertical corn plants provided support for the beans, allowing them to climb upwards. The beans in turn provided nitrogen for the soil. The squash grew horizontally along the ground, preventing the growth of weeds and deterring pests. The three crops benefited each other.

In 1621, Squanto (ca. 1580–1622), a Patuxet Native American Indian, may have changed the course of history by an act of generosity. Squanto's instructions in maize cultivation were responsible for the survival of the pilgrims, who were unprepared for the harsh winters of New England. Over the next decades, the European settlers learned to use the plant in many ways. Corn provided them with ready-to-eat food and fodder for livestock. It was fermented into whiskey. Without corn, the early American pioneers would not have been able to keep pushing west with such vigor.

Corn spread throughout the North American continent in the nineteenth century. The opening of the Erie Canal in 1825 and the defeat of the Sauk, Fox, and Kickapoo Native Americans in the Black Hawk War in 1832 opened up new lands for massive corn cultivation. Corn became big business in the United States by the mid-1800s. A region of the United States, mostly in Iowa and Illinois, but also including parts of Indiana, Minnesota, South Dakota, Nebraska, Kansas, Missouri, and Ohio, became known as the Corn Belt.

Nutritional Aspects of Corn

Corn is nutritionally quite imperfect. It is very low in two essential amino acids: tryptophan and lysine. There is some niacin in corn, but it is "bound" to glucose and proteins. If corn is simply heated and eaten, the niacin in the corn will not be absorbed. In the Americas, before the arrival of the Europeans, corn was an important part of the diet, yet, pre-Columbian and pre-Hispanic populations did not suffer from pellagra. This was due to the ways in which corn was grown and prepared. First, as we saw above, maize was usually grown along with other plants. The "three sisters" was an ingenious agricultural system that helped each plant to grow and also resulted in a diet with a variety of foods. This meant that the Indians were eating food with a fairly complete amino acid and vitamin profile. Second, corn was prepared with alkaline substances, such as ashes or lime. For example, in Mexico, tortillas have always been made using lime solutions. The lime forms a basic, or alkali, solution, which softens the kernel and "frees" some of the niacin so that it is available for absorption once eaten. Corn grown without accompanying plants or not prepared with alkali solutions has calories but no available niacin.

LIME

Lime is a mineral in which calcium is combined with oxygen to form calcium oxide. Calcium oxide has many functions, including "nixtamalization." This is a Spanish borrowing from the Aztec language. It refers to the process of soaking maize in limewater. As a result of nixtamalization, the protein and vitamins in maize become more available.

PELLAGRA: THE ILLNESS OF THE FOUR DS

Pellagra in Europe: A "Disgusting" Disease Blamed on Moldy Corn

Pellagra is the disease resulting from lack of niacin. The person ill with pellagra is known as a "pellagrin." Pellagrins develop scaly red skin on sun-exposed areas of their body. They develop profuse diarrhea and become confused or irritable. Severe cases of the illness result in death. Pellagra is known as the illness of the four Ds: dermatitis, diarrhea, dementia, and death.

The explorers of America took corn back to Europe. Once corn crossed the Atlantic Ocean, it became a major food for sharecroppers in Spain, Italy, and France because it was easy to grow and very productive. Populations increased in areas where corn was introduced. However, corn was grown and treated in Europe in a way that was quite different from how it was grown in America. The corn was not treated with lime, and it was not grown and eaten with squash and beans. In some populations, it came to make up most of the diet. The introduction of corn to Europe meant the introduction of a diet deficient in niacin.

The first description of pellagra came, perhaps suitably, from a Spaniard. Don Gasper Casál described the illness in 1735. He noted the malady among the poorest peasants of the Asturias in northwestern Spain who had diets consisting mostly of maize. The peasants called it *mal de la rosa* because of the skin rash. Casál was impressed by these skin changes and thought that it was a kind of leprosy. He wrote that he had never seen "a more disgusting indigenous disease."[2] The rash sometimes forms a circular lesion around the neck, and this is now known as "Casál's necklace." He described diarrhea and mental disturbances and thought that the illness might be due to spoiled corn.

The term "pellagra" (meaning "rough skin" in Italian) was first used by the Italian physician Francesco Frapoli. In 1771 he described the illness that appeared in Italian field laborers:

> . . . the color of their skin changes suddenly to red, like erysipelas and sometimes reddish spots (which the peasants call "The Rose") appear upon the epidermis and frequently small tubercles of varied color rise up; then the skin becomes dry, the surrounding coats burst, the affected skin falls in white scales just like bran: finally the hands, feet, chest, rarely even the face, and other parts of the body

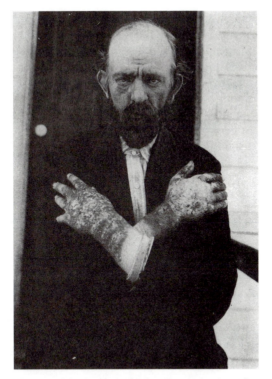

This man has the typical "glove" presentation of
pellagra. Courtesy of the Waring Historical Library,
MUSC, Charleston, S.C.

exposed to the sun become repulsively disfigured . . . the disease rages recur-
rently until at length the skin no longer desquamates but becomes wrinkled, thick-
ened and full of fissures. Then for the first time the patients begin to have trouble
in the head, fear, sadness, wakefulness and vertigo, mental stupor bordering on
fatuity, hypochondria, fluxes from the bowels, and sometimes to suffer from
mania, then the strength of the body fails, especially in the calves and thighs and
they begin to lose motion of those parts almost entirely, to emaciate in the highest
degree, to be seized with a colliquative diarrhoea most resistant to all remedies
and consumed with a ghastly wasting, they approach the last extremity.[3]

The pellagrins were often sharecroppers who were poor farmers with few
resources and little or no cash.

SHARECROPPING

Sharecropping is a system of agriculture that has existed in many different cultures
over many years. Sharecroppers agree to farm a certain plot of land in exchange
for a share of the crops they raise. The sharecropper often is in debt to the land-
owner and lives in poverty and misery.

Pellagra had sprung up in Europe after the introduction of corn and was more common among populations that ate more corn products. Poor people were often forced by circumstances to eat corn that had become moldy. It was natural, therefore, to wonder if corn itself, or moldy corn, caused the illness. There were other theories having nothing to do with corn. Some argued that because the populations suffering from pellagra were sometimes inbred, there must be a hereditary element to the illness. Others noted that because the pellagrins often lived in unsanitary conditions and close to one another, it was likely that pellagra was contagious.

Pellagra in the United States in the Twentieth Century: Common in Insane Asylums

The first case of pellagra in the United States was reported in a poor farmer in 1902. Only four years later, in 1906, eighty-eight patients at Mount Vernon Insane Hospital in Alabama were reported to be ill with pellagra. More than half died. A poor diet was blamed because the food at the hospital consisted mostly of cornmeal or cornmeal-derived products, all of which were filthy and infested with insects. Pellagra was reported in other institutions as well. Was it because of the poor food? There were other possible causes for pellagra appearing in the asylums. Perhaps people ill with pellagra were admitted to these asylums because of the illness itself, or perhaps it was not necessarily more common but just more evident because nurses and physicians in these institutions recorded health problems.

The person who did the most work with respect to pellagra and asylums in the South was James Woods Babcock (1856–1922). He had trained in medicine at Harvard Medical School and in psychiatry at McLean Hospital, both in Massachusetts, and had then returned to his native South Carolina. He became director of the South Carolina State Hospital for the Insane in 1891. Babcock was an energetic man with many accomplishments. He was quick to recognize the seriousness of pellagra.

Babcock and the South Carolina State Board of Health coordinated the first National Conference on Pellagra at the State Hospital for the Insane in Columbia, South Carolina, in November 1909. At this conference it was clear that theories about the cause of pellagra abounded in the United States just as they did in Europe. Many physicians saw it as an infectious disease brought to the country by recent immigrants. This was a time of rapid immigration from eastern and southern Europe, and blaming problems on immigrants was not uncommon. Pellagra was common in Italy; perhaps Italian immigrants brought the "pellagra germ" with them. Other physicians blamed pellagra on the buffalo gnat. Yet others observed that often several members of the same family became ill with pellagra and concluded that the illness was hereditary.

The disease seemed to be becoming more common, and the fear of "catching" pellagra grew. Physicians and nurses at Johns Hopkins in Baltimore, for example, were not allowed to say the word in case it terrified others.

Many hospitals at the time refused to admit pellagrins. The skin manifestations of the illness caused people to describe the pellagrins as "filthy" and "loathsome." Patients with pellagra were shunned. In 1911, pellagra was the leading cause of death in asylums.

Many remedies were tried, including arsenic. The theory was that arsenic would combat the fungus on the spoiled corn that was causing the illness. Arsenic was sometimes given as salvarsan, the treatment developed by Paul Ehrlich for syphilis. Both syphilis and pellagra were associated with skin problems, so it seemed natural to try treatment that worked for syphilis for pellagra. Salvarsan would have made the pellagrins much more ill without being helpful.

Some physicians did attribute the illness to poor nutrition. Fleming Mant Sandwith (1853–1918) was an English physician working in Egypt. He saw pellagra in the fellahin, peasants of the Upper Nile, who ate diets consisting mostly of corn. At the second National Pellagra Conference held in South Carolina in October 1912, Sandwith suggested that pellagra was caused by something missing in the diet. At the same time, Casimir Funk in London suggested that pellagra was a deficiency disease similar to scurvy and beriberi. (Funk almost discovered the cure for pellagra a year later.)

The theory that pellagra was caused by diet was not popular. Despite the prevalence of pellagra in psychiatric institutions where the food was acknowledged to be appalling, the leading theory continued to be that pellagra was an infectious illness. This theory was bolstered by the observation that, as noted above, the damaged skin in pellagrins was somewhat similar to that seen in leprosy and syphilis. Both of these illnesses were known to be infectious. If pellagra was indeed an infectious illness, the argument was that perhaps it spread among asylum inmates thus accounting for the high numbers of mentally ill people ill with pellagra.

Infectious diseases were common in the South. Indeed, much progress was being made at the time with respect to the widespread problem of anemia in the South by focusing on one infectious illness—hookworm infestation. The hookworm became imbedded in the bowel and caused blood loss in the infected person. Physicians believed that pellagra would turn out to be yet another infectious illness, similar to leprosy, syphilis, or hookworm.

The U.S. Public Health Service (USPHS) Sends Goldberger to Investigate

Because of the severity and great number of cases of pellagra, the federal government became involved. Dr. Joseph Goldberger was assigned the problem of pellagra. Goldberger (1874–1929), the youngest of six, was born in the Carpathian Mountains in the Austro-Hungarian Empire. His father, Samuel, was a shepherd who immigrated to the United States after a plague outbreak killed his sheep. Samuel became a grocer and raised his family in the Lower East Side of New York City. The family was poor. Joseph enrolled at City College, determined at first to become an engineer, but changed his mind and entered medical school. He did not do well in private practice and joined the U.S. Marine Hospital Service, which later became the USPHS.

Goldberger was an experienced and intrepid public health doctor who had done much fieldwork with infectious illnesses, including yellow fever, dengue, typhus, hookworm, and diphtheria. He had traveled to Mexico and Cuba to study yellow fever and had become ill with this terrible illness. He had done some "covert medical surveillance" in Mexico, trying to determine how conscientious the officials were in inspecting for yellow fever. He developed dengue in Brownsville, Texas, in 1907. Three years later he fell ill with typhus in Mexico City. Goldberger had also worked with hookworm infestations. He investigated a diphtheria outbreak in Detroit and discovered that a bacteriologist there had been making up data. This was a superb background for his work in pellagra. He had mastered many skills of the "shoe-leather epidemiologist." He had learned—painfully and personally—the characteristics of infectious or contagious illnesses. He had learned that there is no substitute for being "on the ground" to figure out the causes of an illness and not blindly to trust official reports. Goldberger was expected, by the USPHS and himself, to find the infectious cause of pellagra.

Goldberger traveled to the South in early 1914 and visited institutions and communities where pellagra was common. Goldberger saw that attendants and nursing staff in orphanages and asylums spent many hours a day in fairly close contact with the pellagrins yet rarely became ill themselves. This observation was not new, but Goldberger understood its significance. This was not the pattern of an infectious illness. His previous experience with these illnesses had been that medical personnel, including investigators, often became ill with the disease they were treating or studying.

A famous description of the food of the southern poor was the "three Ms"—meat (pork fatback), meal (cornmeal), and molasses. This food was cheap, easy to cook, filling, and tasty. Goldberger became convinced that this atrocious diet was the problem. In June 1914 he wrote a report outlining his theory of the cause of pellagra. The report was not well received. Physicians in the South assured him that this obvious idea had already been considered and rejected. "Look," for example, he was told, "at the Georgia State Sanitarium in Milledgeville. We have asked staff and patients what they eat, and we have the reports: staff and patients eat the same food, but only the patients become ill." Goldberger knew from his earlier work that secondhand reports were not always reliable. He had the good sense to visit the sanitarium. There he saw that what was widely reported was not entirely true. Similar food was *delivered* to staff and patients, but not all *received* good quality food. There was little supervision, and, as a result, the stronger and healthier patients took the choice food, and the weak and ill patients got the leftover food. The staff ate before the patients, so they took the best food; they also had the money and freedom to supplement their diet with food that they purchased from outside the hospital. Goldberger remained certain that food was the key to understanding pellagra.

Goldberger then performed a trial. He arranged for improved diets in two orphanages in Jackson, Mississippi, and in one building of the asylum at Milledgeville, Georgia. He provided fresh milk, meat, and eggs to the orphans and patients. Nothing else was changed. As long as the improved diet was provided, there were no new cases of pellagra. Some patients who recovered from pellagra also recovered from their psychiatric illness and were able to leave the asylum. Once the funding ran out, the old diet was restored, and cases of pellagra again appeared. However, those who believed in an infectious etiology were still not persuaded. A definitive experiment was needed.

The Rankin Farm Experiment

In a famous and controversial experiment, Goldberger arranged for a study at the Rankin State Prison Farm near Jackson, Mississippi. Once again, just as at Bilibid Prison in the Philippines, prisoners proved to be appealing subjects for researchers. Although Mississippi was the state worst hit by pellagra, there were no reports of pellagra in any Mississippi prisons. Indeed, the prisoners seemed to have a better diet than other poor or institutionalized Southerners. Why then use a Mississippi prison? Goldberger chose to do an experiment on the Rankin Farm prisoners in part because of a good working relationship with Earl Brewer, governor of Mississippi. Brewer and Goldberger told about eighty Rankin inmates that if they volunteered to eat a traditional southern diet for about six months and, therefore, run the risk of developing pellagra, they would get full pardons. Brewer and Goldberger selected twelve volunteers. This was a mixed group. Seven were convicted murderers serving life terms. Two were wealthy brothers, serving time for embezzlement after their bank had failed. The brothers were friends of the governor.

In April 1915 the convict volunteers were housed in a scrupulously clean building separated from the other prisoners. They were fed a highly controlled diet. Breakfast consisted of biscuits, fried mush, grits, brown gravy, cane syrup, and coffee. Lunch included corn bread, collards, sweet potatoes, grits, and syrup. Supper was similar to lunch. The usual Rankin prison diet was better in that it contained meat of some sort at all meals, buttermilk, peas, and beans. Prisoners on the experimental diet became ill and weak within two weeks of beginning the diet. The prisoners hated the diet, yet this diet was the standard diet of the southern poor. By the fifth month of the study, in September 1915, six of the volunteers had developed dermatitis and "nervous and gastro-intestinal symptoms." Other physicians confirmed that in five of these prisoners, these changes were consistent with the diagnosis of pellagra. The experiment had succeeded. Goldberger had induced pellagra by feeding otherwise healthy men a diet lacking fresh milk, meat, and vegetables. In retrospect, the prisoners were probably also suffering from other dietary deficiency syndromes, such as riboflavin deficiency, but the point had been made: the poor diet common in the South caused pellagra.

Goldberger's Work Is Disparaged, and His Theory Is Rejected

This experiment was criticized at the time from every angle. The secrecy of the experiment was deplored. Some thought that the prisoners were being treated too harshly, and others claimed that the prisoners were being treated too leniently. Governor Brewer was accused of arranging the whole experiment to "spring" his two friends from prison. Skeptical physicians pointed out that the convicts might have been weakened by the poor diet and that this made them more susceptible to the real cause of pellagra, which was probably infectious.

Why was there opposition to Goldberger's theory? There was medical and popular excitement in the late 1800s and early 1900s about the advances in bacteriology. The microbiologists, with their microscopes, culture plates, and rapidly developing laboratory expertise, were at the forefront of medical knowledge. Goldberger, himself an expert in infectious illnesses, changed his focus from microorganisms to food after visiting the South. His ability to do this at a time when bacteriology was in its ascendancy was comparable with the nimblemindedness of Grijns, Fraser, Stanton, and Strong in Southeast Asia a decade earlier. To us, this ability seems praiseworthy. To physicians and scientists of the time, it seemed wrongheaded.

There were other problems. Wickliffe Rose (1862–1931) was an administrator for the Rockefeller philanthropies and involved in supporting public health initiatives. He directed the crusade against hookworm. He noted that there was often conflict between public health and physicians. He blamed this on the self-interest of the physicians: "A physician has to make a living but that depends on the prevalence of disease. Insofar as this function (prevention) is successful it diminishes the prevalence of disease and therefore diminishes his work and his income."[4] Whether or not this cynicism was justified, it is certain that physicians would be offended by this attitude. Goldberger was a European immigrant, raised in the North, supported by the federal government, who, uninvited by the South, suggested that the southern diet was faulty. Physicians in the South perceived the physicians and administrators from the North as interfering intruders who treated them with contempt and condescension. Eijkman was mocked by his fellow researchers and Goldberger criticized by his fellow physicians. The lot of an original thinker is not easy.

Goldberger's Filth Parties

Goldberger, innovative and determined, had an idea. He was a fair man and just as demanding of himself and colleagues as he was of prisoners. He also was quite accustomed to the risk of developing the disease that he studied. To further establish the dietary rather than infectious nature of pellagra, Goldberger arranged "filth parties." This is a liberal use of the word "party." He tested the contagion theory of pellagra by attempting to transmit the illness by administering secretions or actual excreta of pellagrins or injections of pellagrous blood into healthy subjects. He used volunteers, including other physicians, himself, and his wife. The experiments went on for two months, and although some of the volunteers developed unpleasant side effects such as diarrhea and pain at the site of blood injections, no one developed pellagra. Goldberger was a member of every group. He swallowed sodium bicarbonate with the capsules so that no one could say that his stomach acid had killed the putative infectious agent. At the end of these experiments, Goldberger wrote, "We had our final 'filth party'—Wheeler, Sydenstricker and I—this noon. If anyone can get pellagra that way, we three should certainly have it good and hard. It's the last time. Never again."[5]

The inclusion of his wife among the "volunteers" was unusual. In an account that she wrote years later, she wrote that she had insisted on being a volunteer, "The men would not consent to my swallowing the pills, but I was given by hypodermic in the abdomen an injection of the blood of a woman dying of pellagra. This was an act of faith; it took no courage."[6] Mary Goldberger was too modest. The injection of seven cubic centimeters of blood into her stomach was so upsetting that one nurse who watched this fled from the room crying. Did the experimenters think it more proper to inject a woman with the blood of a woman? Why was swallowing thought to be worse than being injected? The injection was in fact more dangerous than swallowing but somehow less objectionable. These "parties" would probably have had as much trouble being approved today as the Rankin farm studies because of the risks to the subjects. Because of Goldberger's past experience, he must have seen this risk of illness as just part of the quotidian nature of his work.

PHYSICIANS AND SELF-EXPERIMENTATION

Other physicians had tried proving their theories of illnesses by conducting experiments on themselves. The most famous example is John Hunter (1728–1793), who, in trying to investigate venereal diseases, injected his own genitals with pus from an ill man. He developed symptoms of syphilis and gonorrhea and became convinced that the two were the same illness. This thoroughly confused the venereal disease field for some time.

About a century before Goldberger's filth parties, a medical student, Stubbins Ffirth, was studying yellow fever at the University of Pennsylvania. To determine whether or not the illness was contagious, "he injected himself with blood, urine, sweat, black vomit, and other material from yellow fever victims. He then swallowed this material along with all manner of other repulsive substances taken from patients dying of yellow fever."[7] He never became ill. This experiment was actually misleading because yellow fever is contagious.

More recently, Barry Marshall (1951–) won a Nobel Prize by swallowing *Helicobacter pylori* in order to establish the cause of gastric ulcers. Self-experimentation does not guarantee valid results. Hunter and Stubbins Ffirth set back their fields. Goldberger and Marshall, in contrast, because of their experiments, moved medical science forward.

Goldberger may have been one of the few physicians to have his wife be a subject in these experiments. The difference between the outcomes of Goldberger's two studies with "volunteers" was clear. The prison volunteers were exposed to the usual southern diet and became ill. The medical volunteers were exposed to pellagra itself—and stayed well. Taken together, the results pointed, once again, to poor nutrition as a cause of pellagra.

Goldberger described these findings at a medical meeting in Atlanta, Georgia. Opposition to the Northerner from the federal government continued. The southern physicians attending the meeting were outraged at the idea that he was targeting the southern diet as a cause of this illness. A director of a pellagra hospital fumed, "[Goldberger's] advice to discard all drugs and other means other than diet has cast a pall of gloom over our fair Southland and our cemeteries are blooming as do fields of grain after beneficent summer showers . . . physicians all over the South are following his teachings implicitly, crucifying their patients upon a cross of error."[8] The angry director was being disingenuous because he had no treatment for pellagra. He was probably himself helping the southern cemeteries to bloom. In any event, Goldberger had not convinced his colleagues. Moreover, a privately funded commission had surveyed diets in the South and concluded that there was no connection between pellagra and diet. Vedder in the Philippines, who had played a significant part in defeating beriberi and who had a wide ranging interest in nutritional deficiency, had reviewed this commission's findings and doubted their conclusions. He supported Goldberger but was far from the field of conflict. Yet more work was needed.

The Seven-Cotton-Mill Village Survey

In the spring of 1916 Goldberger began yet another line of investigation into pellagra. He decided to survey communities to try to determine a link between diet and pellagra. Why repeat surveys that had already been done? Goldberger's idea was simple and powerful. He would repeat the survey but do it meticulously. As he had learned many times before, reports from others could be misleading. He and his team, with George A. Wheeler and Edgar Sydenstricker (members of the filth parties), organized house-to-house canvases of seven cotton-mill villages in South Carolina. Wheeler and Sydenstricker were probably happier with their new assignment.

Goldberger chose these villages because pellagra was common there. Mill owners, just like those who ran institutions, provided their workers with food that was cheap and easy to buy, transport, and store. Cotton-mill villages were notorious for the poor health of their workers. To understand this, we will review briefly the history of southern industry as it relates to cotton.

Pellagra: The Cotton Connection and Child Labor

Pellagra flourished in the mill villages of the South because of certain agricultural practices. The warm climate, long growing season, abundant rainfall, and fertile soil might have meant that a multitude of crops could have been grown in this region. Instead, monocultural practices—growing one crop only over large areas—developed. Monoculture is efficient because it is easier to use specialized forms of labor and/or machinery to plant, tend, and harvest just one crop and is often used for cash crops. Cash crops are those sold by the farmer to others for cash, rather than crops grown for use by the farmer. The first cash crops raised in the South were tobacco and cotton.

Before the 1700s, cotton and wool were processed into cloth in the household using foot-powered spinning wheels and hand looms. The first step was the formation of thread. Fibers were spun into thread using the spinning wheel. Cloth is made from two different types of thread: warp and weft. Warp threads are strong and run lengthwise through the material, and in the past were made of wool. Weft threads are weaker and cross the warp, and were made of cotton. The threads were woven together on a loom to form cloth. The job of spinning and weaving was tedious and slow, but changed with the inventions of machines in the 1700s.

Richard Arkwright (1732–1792), an Englishman, invented the spinning, or water, frame in 1767. This frame produced strong threads from yarn. Arkwright's invention allowed cotton to be strong enough to form the warp threads for the first time. Cloth could now be made entirely of cotton and in a mechanized way. This is one of the inventions that began the Industrial Revolution. Foot-powered spinning wheels and hand looms in the home were replaced by water-powered machines located in factories. For many decades, American cotton was sent across the Atlantic and processed in the textile mills in England. The details of the English machinery were kept in great secrecy. Blueprints were scarce and guarded zealously. Skilled textile mechanics were forbidden to emigrate. Samuel Slater (1768–1835) of Belper, Derbyshire, worked at the Arkwright-Strutt mills for eight years. He learned how these new machines worked and, as all employees had to do, swore never to reveal the trade secrets.

Slater slipped away from Arkwright-Strutt and immigrated to the United States in 1789. He had no papers or blueprints. He went into business with Moses Brown (1738–1836) in Pawtucket, Rhode Island. They recreated the Arkwright-Strutt mills and their machinery, relying on Slater's memory. Along with the new machinery, Slater introduced a new way of working. In 1803 he built a mill village, Slatersville. This village housed the mill, homes for the workers, and a company store. Many of the employees were children. Slater is known as the father of the American Industrial Revolution, or the father of the American factory system. In England, he is remembered as "Slater the traitor."

The process of preparing the cotton was becoming mechanized at the same time as the process of preparing the cloth. Eli Whitney (1765–1825), an American, invented (or improved) the cotton gin in 1793. The gin mechanized the tedious and time-consuming task of separating the sticky seeds and seed pods from the cotton fibers. Cotton became one of the first cash crops to be associated with mechanical means of production. Whitney's gin has been celebrated as one of the greatest inventions of the time.

Whitney became embroiled in a nasty struggle about who had actually invented the gin. He spent more time and energy on this struggle than on developing the machine. In 1806, nine years after Whitney's invention, Judge William Johnson in Georgia decided that Whitney did indeed deserve to be known as inventor of the cotton gin. Johnson put the invention of the gin into context by explaining, from the point of view of the South, the social implications of Whitney's work:

> The whole interior of the Southern States was languishing, and its inhabitants emigrating for want of some object to gain their attention, and employ their industry, when the invention of this machine at once opened views to them, which set the whole country in active motion. From childhood to age it has presented to us a lucrative employment. Individuals who were depressed with poverty, and sunk in idleness, have suddenly risen in wealth and respectability . . . Our sister States, also, participate in the benefits of this invention; for, besides affording the raw material for their manufactures, the bulkiness and quantity of the articles afford a valuable employment for their shipping.[9]

The good judge's interest in employment for children is interesting and not unusual for the time. At the end of the eighteenth century, most Americans were farmers. This was celebrated by some, such as Thomas Jefferson (1743–1826), but lamented by others, such as Alexander Hamilton (1755–1804), who worried that America could never compete with Europe. Hamilton wrote that women and children were more useful when employed in manufacturing establishments.[10]

Just as the secrets of the mills were bound to move from Belper, Derbyshire, to Pawtucket, Rhode Island, so the New England mills and mill villages also were certain to move south. There were obvious economic advantages to placing cotton-mill villages in the South rather than in New England. The southern mills were closer to the cotton itself, and labor in the South was willing and cheap.

Women and children made up most of the mill workforce and were paid poorly, but work in the mills was better than hot and back-breaking work in the fields. Families moved from farms to mill villages. The cotton mills were part of an economic revival in the South and the beginning of southern industrial development. The South was then poverty-stricken, and jobs for women and children were welcomed. The employment of children, as noted by Judge Johnson and Alexander Hamilton, was seen not as exploitation but as a social good. Mill owners were delighted to have child employees. Children were quicker than adults to learn how to work the machinery. They could be paid less. The consequences for the children were mixed. They made money for themselves and their families, but they worked long hours, sometimes with dangerous machinery, were deprived of education or recreation, and were fed badly. In the southern states, eleven-hour workdays six

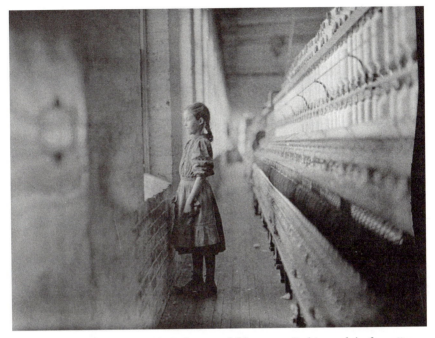

This eleven-year-old girl is typical of young children recruited to work in the cotton mills. She had been working for over a year. The picture was taken in 1908. Photograph by Lewis W. Hine. National Archives (102-LH-249).

days a week were legal, even for children. (Other consequences of child labor will be reviewed in Chapter 6.)

Workers in the mills were like sharecroppers in that their lives were controlled by others. The mill owners organized housing and provided company stores. Sometimes the company stores maintained wage accounts and subtracted the cost of food before giving the workers their wages. Wages were low, and the housing and food that the companies provided were of poor quality.

The millworkers did not have the land, time, or energy to tend gardens or to raise any livestock. Much of their diet consisted of cornmeal products. Corn could be grown in parts of America with relatively short growing seasons, such as the Midwest. Therefore, cotton—more particular in where it chose to grow well—was grown in the South, and corn was grown in the Midwest. Food for the poor in the South was corn grown in the Midwest.

In the early twentieth century, a machine known as the Beall Degerminator was devised. Using this machine and others like it, corn from the Midwest was milled. During this process the germ and oil were removed, which made the cornmeal easier to store and easier to ship by rail to the South; this is because the corn kernel contains a small amount of oil around the germ, which can become rancid. Another result of the milling process was that the corn also became less nutritious. Once again, as with rice in Southeast Asia, milling is a double-edged sword. The milling results in better-tasting food that lasts longer, but it comes at a price: vitamin depletion.

The cotton monoculture and improvement in cotton processing and cloth manufacture stimulated southern industry but left the diet of the southern cotton-mill worker in the hands of the midwestern Corn Belt farmers and the maws of the Beall Degerminator.

The Survey Takes Place

Women and children working in the cotton mills were concentrated in the villages and had little access to transportation. As with Fraser and Stanton's road builders and Strong's Bilibid prisoners, this density of population and lack of mobility may have been miserable for the people involved, but it was a boon for researchers. Goldberger's surveyors visited homes in these villages every two weeks to obtain accurate data about diet and to determine the incidence of pellagra. This was painstaking, tedious, and delicate work. The surveyors were strangers who were asking highly intrusive questions of people. Eventually, they came up with answers that were a closer approximation to the truth than were the findings of the earlier and more rapidly done survey. The quality of the research findings was, as is always the case, only as good as the quality of the work that went into the surveys. Shortcuts made the work easy and useless.

The surveyors believed that they were obtaining accurate reports from the villagers about what they were eating. But were they? They needed to confirm or validate their results. The surveyors cleverly took advantage of the peculiar source of food in these mill villages and cross-checked their data with records in village stores. Company or village stores may not have provided good quality food, but they provided good quality data for this survey. By repeated home visits and respectful questioning and then by checking their findings against the store records, Goldberger's team came up with a clear picture of the diet of the people in the seven cotton-mill villages and its relationship to pellagra:

- Pellagra was both more common and less serious than had been recognized previously. The surveyors picked up mild cases that otherwise would have been missed.
- It was more common in people who ate little meat and milk because of poverty.
- Pellagra did not increase with the amount of corn that the villagers ate. The cause of pellagra was not what the pellagrins ate, but what they did not eat. Corn displaced other, higher quality, foods. Someone who ate a lot of corn would not become ill with pellagra as long as he or she was also eating other foods.
- It was predominantly a disease of children.

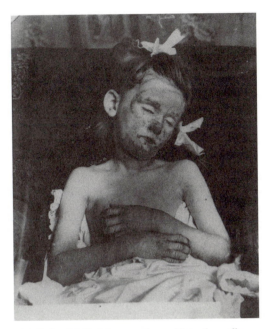

This little girl died from pellagra. Note the pellagra
rash over her lower arms and neck. Courtesy of the
Waring Historical Library, MUSC, Charleston, S.C.

In other words, pellagra was a common, chronic illness that affected the
poor, particularly their children, who ate too little nutritious food. Without a
systematic door-to-door survey, these findings could not have been made.
Goldberger concluded that pellagra was a malady related to southern poverty. This conclusion was similar to that of the United Nations beriberi
experts who saw that disease just as much as a disease of poverty as of thiamine deficiency.

Dogs with Black Tongue Are Treated with Yeast; Yeast Is Given to Refugees from the Mississippi Floods

In the late 1920s, Goldberger continued his work with pellagra by working
with dogs. He was lucky to find a good animal model of pellagra in the canine
illness "black tongue." Hunting dogs were likely to become ill with black
tongue when their diet was mostly cornbread. Owners of hunting dogs fed
their dogs this diet to make them lose weight so that they could be swifter.

Goldberger suspected that lack of protein was the problem in both pellagra and black tongue. In 1901, Hopkins had discovered the essential amino
acid tryptophan, a building block for protein. Rats died within two weeks
if their diet did not include tryptophan. Goldberger had successfully treated
pellagra in orphanages and asylums by adding milk or meat, both of which
contained tryptophan. Perhaps lack of tryptophan caused pellagra.

Goldberger arranged for dogs to be fed experimental diets consisting of cornbread and molasses to see whether he could cause black tongue. This became known as the "Goldberger diet." His plan was to cause black tongue and then experiment with different foods to see which would cure the disease, but as the dogs became ill, they developed sore mouths, which made it difficult for them to eat. This complicated the experiment. Goldberger wanted to make sure that he was seeing the effects of their restricted diet and not just starvation. He consulted with experts. A veterinarian advised him to give the dogs yeast. Brewer's yeast was used in those days as a veterinary panacea and appetite enhancer; Goldberger followed this advice and added yeast to the diets of the dogs.

The dogs ate well but, annoyingly, did not become ill with black tongue. The experiment had hit a roadblock. Then, it made sense to him—yeast was not a problem, it was the answer. Just as unpolished rice cured Eijkman's chickens of polyneuritis, so did brewer's yeast cure Goldberger's dogs of black tongue. Brewer's yeast is an excellent source of B vitamins. However, brewer's yeast does not contain tryptophan, which is what Goldberger had suspected to be the anti-pellagra substance.

YEAST

Yeasts are single-celled fungi related to mushrooms. They have been used for fermentation and baking for thousands of years. Louis Pasteur discovered that yeasts ferment sugars to form the alcohol present in wine. Nutritional yeast, *Saccaromyces cerevisiae*, is grown specifically for its nutritional value because it produces many proteins and vitamins. Yeast, in the form of marmite, was also used by Lucy Wills in treating pregnant anemic women. This is discussed in the chapter about Vitamins B9 and B12.

Despite the lack of tryptophan in yeast, Goldberger decided to use it for people ill with pellagra. He gave pellagrins in asylums yeast and saw that they got better. He was in the middle of organizing a series of trials to formally show the benefits of yeast when an "opportunity" to use it occurred. In 1927, after months of above-normal rainfall in the Midwest, the Mississippi overflowed its banks. This famous and disastrous Mississippi flood was also associated with drought and infestation, all of which led to crop failure. Thousands of refugees became malnourished, and as many as 50,000 people developed pellagra.

Goldberger traveled to the affected areas in Arkansas, Louisiana, Mississippi, and Tennessee. He advised the Red Cross to add brewer's yeast to its food rations. Within weeks, people with pellagra were cured, and new cases of pellagra were prevented. Without yeast, the devastation caused by the flood would have been far worse. Goldberger died in 1929, eight years before the actual cure for pellagra (and solution to the tryptophan-yeast puzzle) was found.

Summary of Goldberger's Work

Goldberger achieved much and mastered many disciplines in his work with pellagra. He had made the correct decision to leave his job as a private practitioner to become a public health researcher. By improving the diet in institutions, he cured the disease. By restricting the diet in a prison population, he caused it. His community surveys led him to understand and emphasize the socioeconomic causes of this nutritional deficiency. He found an animal model of the disease in the canine illness "black tongue" and discovered that yeast could cure the illness. He introduced the use of yeast as a nutritional supplement for humans to treat pellagra. Goldberger established that pellagra was a nutritional deficiency disease, similar to beriberi, rather than an infectious illness. Goldberger began his career in public health as an expert in infectious diseases and ended it as an expert in the three Ps: politics, poverty, and pellagra.

Nicotinic Acid: A Cheap Photographic Chemical and a Vitamin

Conrad Elvehjem (1901–1962) was a researcher at the University of Wisconsin with impeccable credentials for work with vitamins. As a youngster growing up in Wisconsin, he learned about Babcock's early experiments while still in grade school. He wrote his senior thesis with Steenbock, the discoverer of Vitamin D. He had also studied at Cambridge in the United Kingdom.

Elvehjem induced black tongue in dogs by feeding them the Goldberger diet. He then cured this illness by supplementing their diet with a substance derived from a liver extract, originally known as vitamin G (G for Goldberger). This substance turned out to be nicotinic acid.

The story of how Elvehjem finally made this discovery is complicated. Nicotinic acid was synthesized in 1873 and used in photography. No one thought of it as having anything to do with food or health until German scientists showed that nicotinic acid occurred in yeast and in rice polishings. In 1913, Casimir Funk went further and showed that nicotinic acid was in the part of yeast and rice polishings that treated beriberi. He thought that nicotinic acid was the cure for beriberi. He was wrong, but he showed that nicotinic acid probably had nutritional value.

Other researchers showed that a type of chemical known as a pyridine could be found in liver extracts. In 1934, Otto Warburg (1883–1970) found nicotinamide, a pyridine closely related to nicotinic acid, in red blood cells. Using Warburg's method, Elvehjem found nicotinamide in liver extracts. He suspected that nicotinamide, or its close relative nicotinic acid, was the anti-pellagra substance. He contacted Eastman-Kodak and obtained pure nicotinic acid and gave it to a dog with black tongue. The dog improved. In 1937, he reported that both nicotinic acid and nicotinamide cured and prevented black tongue.

Pellagra could be cured by yeast, by other dietary improvements such as more protein, or by nicotinic acid—an inexpensive photographic chemical.

The next step was to use this chemical, previously just used in photography, in humans. Physicians first consumed it themselves and noted no ill effects except for a flush. Then, they took the next step. They gave the chemical to pellagrins. Physicians reported success in treating pellagra with nicotinic acid. This achievement was lauded in the *New York Times* in 1938:

> What this success means, the statistics proclaim adequately enough. So far as the United States Public Health Service can determine 400,000 people succumb to pellagra in this country every year—an underestimate. If the diet is not corrected the death rate is as high as 69%. Worse still the mind is affected. Fully 10 per cent of the inmates of our institutions for the mentally afflicted suffer from pellagra.
>
> To restore the victims to health of body and mind by adding the proper food doses of a cheap chemical seems miraculous. . . .[11]

As formerly noted, in 1941, the U.S. Congress recommended the vitamin fortification of bread. Representatives of the baking industry were alarmed, suspecting that if customers knew that bread was fortified with nicotinic acid they would not buy it, thinking that it had been supplemented with nicotine. After consultation with Elvehjem and others, niacin was chosen as a synonym for nicotinic acid. The bakers withdrew their objections.

Why Does Brewer's Yeast Cure Pellagra?

Humans can make niacin from the amino acid tryptophan. However, this synthesis is inefficient. About 60 mg of dietary tryptophan is equivalent to 1 mg of nicotinic acid. Therefore, niacin is still considered a vitamin, that is, an organic substance that must be ingested. Tryptophan, an amino acid, is found in large amounts in many protein-rich foods. This explains why protein-rich foods were helpful in the treatment of pellagra.

NIACIN AND SCHIZOPHRENIA

Three Young Men in England Think about Schizophrenia and Mescaline

Niacin plays a part in the history of psychiatry quite apart from the high prevalence of pellagra in asylums in the past. The story of niacin as a heralded (but eventually disproven) treatment for schizophrenia began when young psychiatrists made a series of biochemical speculations.

SCHIZOPHRENIA

Schizophrenia is a common and severe psychiatric illness. The person with schizophrenia may have delusions, which are fixed and false beliefs, or difficulty with abstract thinking. They may have difficulty beginning or organizing activities. They may hear noises or voices that others do not hear. Many people with schizophrenia are anxious or depressed and have difficulty forming relationships or keeping jobs.

In 1951, John Smythies (a resident at St. George's hospital in London), John Harley-Mason (an organic chemist at Cambridge University), and Humphry Osmond (a physician) (1917–2004) became interested in the experiences of normal volunteers using mescaline, the substance found in the peyote plant that causes hallucinations. They thought that there were some similarities between schizophrenia and mescaline experiences. Mescaline is similar in structure to adrenaline. The three young men wondered if the schizophrenic body or brain might contain an adrenaline-like substance that, just like mescaline, caused hallucinations.

The English psychiatry establishment was not impressed. Osmond decided to get far away from English indifference to his theories and moved to Canada. He became assistant director of the large mental hospital in the remote city of Weyburn, Saskatchewan. This was a fortuitous move for him because he became friendly with the provincial director of psychiatric research, Abram Hoffer, who worked in Saskatoon, Saskatchewan.

Abram Hoffer (1917–) grew up on a farm in Saskatchewan. He worked in a lab adding vitamins to flour in Winnipeg and later received his Ph.D. in agricultural chemistry, studying thiamine in cereals. He then went to medical school and became a psychiatrist. This was an ideal background for someone who would spend much of his life studying vitamins and schizophrenia. Hoffer and Osmond worked together for the next several decades.

Hoffer and Osmond believed that niacin prevented the production of adrenaline and therefore perhaps could prevent hallucinations. They used the vitamin to treat schizophrenic patients in Saskatoon. Patients treated with niacin spent fewer days in the hospital, had fewer readmissions, and fewer suicide attempts than patients treated without the vitamin. It seemed that niacin was an excellent treatment for this hitherto untreatable illness. But, as we shall see with James Lind, it is the job of researchers to doubt their results, and to consider other possibilities. Could the researchers have deceived themselves? Perhaps they chose patients who were less ill, or perhaps their enthusiasm about niacin was what actually helped their patients. In all branches of medicine the placebo effect, or a response to a treatment arising from the patient's hope that the treatment will be helpful, can complicate studies of treatment. Hoffer and Osmond considered, and rejected, the possibility that the less ill patients were treated with niacin, or that there was a marked placebo effect, noting that:

> . . . nicotinic acid patients tended to be sicker than the comparison group for with any new treatment doctors are often loathe to try it upon those they feel will respond well to orthodox measures . . . (most of the patients) were treated by psychiatrists who were indifferent, skeptical, or openly hostile to the whole idea (of niacin treatment). They put their hope in psychotherapy and would only allow their less desirable patients, who seemed unsuitable for psychotherapy, to be included in the nicotinic acid trial . . . [12]

Hoffer and Osmond thought that they were able to be so productive because of their location in Saskatchewan. Osmond had gone there to escape from the rigid and conservative English medical establishment, but it proved to be helpfully far away from the equally rigid and conservative Canadian medical establishment. As is clear from what they wrote above, even in Saskatchewan they encountered physicians who were "indifferent, skeptical, or openly hostile . . ." to their ideas. Hoffer wrote that medical schools with their research and ethics committees would have slowed down his and Osmond's work.

But perhaps their isolation caused them problems, too. They complained that their work was ignored by the academic community. They wondered about this lack of attention and wrote that one reason might have been the "extraordinary proliferation of the phenothiazine derivatives since 1954. Unlike these, niacin is a simple well-known vitamin which can be bought cheaply in bulk and cannot be patented, and there has been no campaign to persuade doctors of its usefulness. . . ."[13]

In other words, pharmaceutical companies promoted their new and expensive drugs while no one promoted niacin because there were no profits to be made from this simple chemical.

Linus Pauling Calls Schizophrenia "Cerebral Pellagra" and Develops a New Theory of "Mental Malnutrition"

The work of Osmond and Hoffer with niacin had a strong influence on the two-time Nobel Prize winner Linus Pauling (1901–1994). Pauling identified sickle-cell anemia as one of the first molecular diseases. (Pauling and his other contributions to vitamins are also discussed in the chapters about vitamins B9, B12, and C.)

Pauling described "*orthomolecular psychiatry*" as the treatment of mental disease by providing the best possible molecular environment for the brain. He argued that the brain was more sensitive to "abnormal molecular concentrations of essential substances" than other organs and suggested that schizophrenia might be due to an unusual need for very large doses of vitamins. Pauling thought that most psychiatric disorders could be traced to a vitamin or other nutrient deficiency to which some people might be extremely sensitive. He coined the term "cerebral pellagra" to describe schizophrenia.

Does Niacin Treat Schizophrenia?

The Canadian Mental Health Association (CMHA) organized a series of studies to test the efficacy of niacin in patients with schizophrenia. The CMHA concluded from these trials that niacin was not helpful and indeed in some cases had "a negative therapeutic effect."[14] An independent two-year study of the effects of nicotinic acid in eighty-six patients with schizophrenia also found no evidence to support its usefulness,[15] and laboratory researchers were unable to find evidence to support the theories of Osmond and Hoffer.

With the negative findings of the CMHA and other trials and no laboratory support, interest in the psychiatric community in the therapeutic effects of niacin has faded.

The question of how Osmond and Hoffer were able to obtain such good responses to niacin will probably remain unanswered. Few physicians today believe that large doses of niacin are helpful in psychiatry.

Hoffer, Niacin, and Cholesterol

In 1955, Hoffer and his colleagues in Saskatchewan discovered that high doses of niacin lowered cholesterol.[16] It was the first substance shown to do this and the first medication shown to reduce heart attacks and to lower long-term mortality rates. It is not commonly used now because it is associated with severe flushes. (These flushes had been experienced by the physicians who took niacin before using it to treat pellagra.)

Perhaps another reason for its relative lack of popularity is similar to what Osmond and Hoffer suspected. It is a vitamin and cannot be patented, so no pharmaceutical companies vigorously promote it.

SUMMARY

Niacin is both a photographic chemical and a vitamin. The Native Americans grew and prepared maize in such a way that they were able to obtain niacin from their food. When corn was grown by Europeans, it was treated in a different way. For 200 years, the corn plant, with its more productive method of photosynthesis, formed the bulk of the diet of many sharecroppers, fellahin, peasants, inhabitants of orphanages and asylums, and cotton-mill workers. As a result, the lives of many of these impoverished people were blighted by the "disgusting" disease of pellagra with its skin rashes, diarrhea, mental problems, and sometimes death. The USPHS expected to find an infectious cause of this illness, but, to the surprise of everyone except Sandwith and Funk, Goldberger found that pellagra was related to poverty and the grinding and relentless efficiency of the corn degerminators. The Native Americans ate corn but were well supplied with niacin. The cotton-mill workers in the South ate cornmeal and became niacin deficient.

The discovery of yeast and liver extracts as a cure for black tongue in dogs led to the discovery of nicotinic acid, a cheap chemical, now known as the vitamin niacin. Psychiatrists hoped that large doses of niacin would cure "cerebral pellagra," more commonly known as schizophrenia, but this has not been shown to be effective. However, one of these psychiatrists was involved in the discovery that niacin lowers cholesterol—an important finding.

4

Deadly Anemia, Sludge, and the Nobel Prize for a Woman: Vitamins B9 (Folate) and B12 (Cobalamin), the Two Anti-anemia Vitamins

Overview

The discoveries of folate (Vitamin B9) and cobalamin (Vitamin B12) are intertwined with the history of hematology—the science of blood. These two vitamins work together (with other factors) to produce red blood cells. Anemia, a disorder in which there are too few red blood cells, develops if there is insufficient folate and/or cobalamin (see Appendix 3).

The discovery of folate involved experiments on dogs in Rochester, New York, and rats and monkeys in Bombay (now Mumbai). A young English doctor working in India studied pregnant women, some of whom died from their anemia. Laboratory work with one monkey changed her approach to this disorder. She cured her patients with Marmite, a pungent English spread made up of spent yeast. Marmite is rich in many B vitamins, including folate. For a short time, folate was named "Wills' factor" after her.

Cobalamin was the last vitamin to be discovered. The illness associated with Vitamin B12 deficiency is pernicious anemia. One physician discovered how to treat this illness by regurgitating his own stomach contents. Pernicious anemia, unlike the other illnesses associated with vitamin deficiencies, is not a nutritional deficiency disorder. In this illness, there is enough Vitamin B12 in the diet, but it is not absorbed properly. Pernicious anemia is an autoimmune illness.

Cobalamin is a large and intricate molecule. Chemists used computers to decipher its three-dimensional structure. An international team, led by a Nobel Prize winner, eventually synthesized it. Microorganisms in muck have been able to make this vitamin, with less fanfare, for billions of years.

Folate (Vitamin B9)

Work in Bombay

A young English doctor working in Bombay (now Mumbai) made key observations that led to the discovery of folate. Dr. Lucy Wills (1888–1964) was born into a wealthy English family. She obtained a double first honors degree in botany and geology from Cambridge University. She did some research in geology, traveled to South Africa, returned to England to attend medical school, and graduated with a degree in medicine from the Royal Free Hospital for Women in London in 1920. She worked in London as a biochemist for eight years and in 1928 was recruited by the Indian Medical Service to work in Bombay. Her patients were desperately ill women with multiple and poorly understood illnesses cared for in overcrowded and underequipped hospitals. Wills' focus of study was megaloblastic or macrocytic anemia in pregnant women (see Appendix 3). Some of these women had as few as 450,000 cells in each cubic milliliter of blood, which is less than one tenth of the normal number of red cells. The anemia in these pregnant women caused heart failure and death.

She took a systematic approach to this problem. She began by searching for infectious causes because some transmittable illnesses, such as malaria or hookworm, cause blood loss. She spent much time examining the stool of anemic women searching for evidence of infection. Nothing much came from this line of investigation. (This is reminiscent of McCollum studying cow dung.)

Then, she considered nutritional causes. With a colleague, Sakuntala Talpade, she surveyed the diets of these women. Bombay was a poor city with a splendidly diverse population. The women belonged to different religions—Hindu, Muslim, Christian, Bene-Israel, and Parsee—and followed different diets. The survey was complicated because income also affected diet. It turned out that the women most likely to become anemic were the poor women, no matter what their religion, who ate the least variety of foods and the fewest vegetables. The poorer women were also more likely to have access only to milk that was watered down or contaminated, so they often boiled their milk. Wills and colleagues suspected that the diets of the anemic women might be low in the recently discovered Vitamins A and/or C.

Marmite and One Monkey

Wills also worked with laboratory animals. She fed the rats the same diet that was available to women in India that was associated with macrocytic anemia, and the monkeys also became anemic. Wills added Vitamins A and C, with no success. This meant that there was a *different* deficiency in their diet. Wills continued working with the rats, but the results became confusing for a couple of reasons. First, laboratory rats are often infected with a type of bacteria, *Bartonella*, which can cause anemia. Second, later work showed that rats have other bacteria in their gut that can make folate. Wills and her team switched to rhesus monkeys. These monkeys were not infected with *Bartonella*, or the folate-making bacteria, so these complications were removed.

Wills fed the monkeys the diet that was associated with macrocytic anemia in the pregnant women, and the monkeys also became anemic. She persuaded one anemic rhesus monkey to eat Marmite. The monkey's anemia disappeared.

MARMITE

The German chemist Justus Liebig, a pioneer in nutrition discussed in the Vitamin A chapter, realized that a byproduct of the brewing process, spent yeast, could be made into a concentrated food product. This yeast extract became known as Marmite. The Marmite Food Company began to produce this in 1902 at Burton-on-Trent in England. Marmite became a popular spread in the United Kingdom and British colonies.

Wills had made monkeys anemic by giving them the same diets as Indian women; then, she treated the women with what had helped one monkey. It is remarkable that she drew conclusions from an experiment with one monkey. It would have been more prudent to repeat the experiment in other monkeys or laboratory animals. Why did she move so quickly to try Marmite in her patients?

Wills was independent and decisive. At a time when few women traveled alone or went to medical school, she had done both. She was about to return to England and may have felt that she had to work very quickly to see if her finding with the monkey had real clinical relevance. The grave illnesses of the women may have spurred her on. Wills treated women with megaloblastic anemia with Marmite or extracts of liver. (The reason for the liver was the work of Whipple and Robscheit to be described later.) She was successful—the women recovered. It seems peculiar that the anti-anemia factor was found in liver and spent yeast. These are not popular foods. Liver must have been particularly offensive to those women who were vegetarian. Marmite has a strong taste, which is delicious to those who have been exposed to it in childhood, but not to others.

Wills returned to England in 1932 and worked with biochemists at the Lister Institute in London to identify the anti-anemic substances present in liver and Marmite. Marmite is rich in B vitamins. Could the anemia have been related to beriberi, the B1 deficiency disease? This seemed unlikely because beriberi was not common in Bombay. Deficiency of a different B vitamin was involved in the anemia of pregnant women.

Wills' observations of the beneficial effects of liver and Marmite changed the way in which anemias were understood and led to the identification of folate as a vitamin needed to make red blood cells. Wills' contribution to medicine was especially noteworthy given the difficult conditions in which she was working. Because of her Bombay work, folate was originally called Wills' factor.

Wills' Factor Is Named Folate and Is Found in Spinach

This unknown factor present in Marmite and liver that could treat some kinds of macrocytic anemias was isolated from spinach, another unpopular food, by scientists at the University of Texas in 1941. It turns out that folates are common in green vegetables. The factor was named folate (*Latin folium,* leaf). One of the scientists who identified folate was Roger Williams. (His older brother, Robert Williams, worked with beriberi for many years and had solved the chemical formula of another B vitamin, thiamine.)

Lederle Laboratories scientists isolated some folate crystals from one and a half tons of liver, determined its structure, synthesized it in August 1943, and began to market it the next year. Then, the process slowed down. There was some hesitation about the use of folate as a supplement. Folate could treat megaloblastic anemia caused by folate deficiency, but this turned out to be rare in the United States. Wills might not have identified folate if she had gone to Boston rather than Bombay. Was there really a market for synthetic folate?

Other concerns arose. In 1947 physicians became aware that folate could also treat, to some extent, the megaloblastic anemia caused by Vitamin B12 deficiency. Far from being helpful, this was actually quite harmful. Some symptoms found in Vitamin B12 deficiency anemia (which will be discussed below) were quite different from those of folate deficiency anemias and consisted of neurological problems. Many physicians thought that folate worsened the neurological signs and symptoms of Vitamin B12 deficiency while "masking" the anemia.[1] The concern was as follows. A physician might treat an anemic Vitamin B12-deficient patient with folate and think that the illness was cured if the anemia responded. Meanwhile, the neurological symptoms of the Vitamin B12 deficiency could be worsening. The situation became more complicated with new discoveries about the beneficial effects of folate.

More about Folate and Pregnancy

Folate deficiency in pregnancy is dangerous. The consequences for the mother, as described in the papers of Lucy Wills, could be a megaloblastic anemia leading to congestive heart failure and death. Several decades later, it was discovered that, for the fetus, low folate causes a different problem. Low folate increases the chance of neural tube defects (NTDs).

NTDs

The neural tube is the embryonic form of the spinal cord. Embryonic cells form a narrow tube, which develops into the brain and spinal cord. The tube is usually closed by about twenty-eight days. In NTDs, the spinal cord does not close completely during the first few weeks of pregnancy. Depending on the degree to which the tube closes, the consequences can range from minor (cosmetic problems) to catastrophic (failure of the brain to develop). Spina bifida is one of the most common forms of NTD. In this disorder, the spinal cord is exposed, usually in the lower back. There may be a variety of problems involving impaired bowel and bladder control and leg weakness.

Several large studies suggested that the addition of folic acid, the synthetic form of folate, to the diets of pregnant women could lower the number of

NTDs. NTDs occur very early in pregnancy, often before the woman knows that she is pregnant. To ensure that all women have enough folate in their diet during the important first month of pregnancy, some countries have decided to add folic acid to common foods.

Manufacturers in the United States have been required since 1998 to add folic acid to many grain products. Grain products (most breads, flours, corn-meal, rice, noodles, and macaroni) were chosen because they are staples for most of the population. There has been ongoing controversy about the supplementation of flour and grains with folate because of the possibility of folate interfering with the diagnosis of Vitamin B12 deficiency. The U.S. Food and Drug Administration chose to supplement flour at a rate that was thought insufficient by some, in terms of diminishing the rate of NTDs, to make sure that Vitamin B12 deficiency anemia would not be overlooked.

Since the folic acid fortification program took effect, fortified foods have become a major source of folic acid in the American diet, and there has been a reduction of between 15 and 50 percent in NTDs in the United States. It is not understood how low folate in the maternal diet increases the chances of NTDs.

COBALAMIN (VITAMIN B12)

Vitamin B12, or cobalamin, was the last vitamin to be discovered. It is the only molecule in the body to contain cobalt. Cobalamin is found in mud or sludge. Despite these undignified origins, its structure is so complicated that the scientists who elucidated its structure were awarded Nobel Prizes. Cobalamin, as well as folate, is involved in the synthesis of red blood cells.

"The Dogs Were Bled . . . to a Hemoglobin Level of about One Third of Their Normal Values . . ."

The history of the discovery of cobalamin begins with pernicious anemia. The adjective "pernicious" comes from the Latin root "nex," meaning "violent," and means highly injurious, destructive, or deadly. Patients with pernicious anemia, until the work to be described below, inevitably died because of the illness.

Physicians working in Rochester and Boston in the early twentieth century began the work that led to the successful treatment of this illness and the discovery of cobalamin. George Hoyt Whipple (1878–1976) and Frieda Robscheit-Robbins (1893–1973) were studying diseases of the blood in Rochester, New York. They bled dogs to make them anemic. This work was not for the fainthearted or for dog lovers:

> [Robscheit-Robbins] took charge of the laboratory and ran it with an iron hand, permitting no deviation from the set program . . . She bled the dogs, trained them to cooperate in the experiments . . . The dogs were bled, by aspiration from the jugular vein, to a hemoglobin level of about one third of their normal

values. This anemia was maintained at a constant level for the duration of the dogs' lives, often as long as five to eight years, by removal of newly formed blood.[2]

After making these dogs anemic, Whipple and Robscheit-Robbins experimented with various ways of treating the anemia. They fed the dogs food from different organs and found that liver was the most effective. This work influenced Lucy Wills in Bombay and also George R. Minot (1885–1950) and William P. Murphy (1892–1987), who were studying pernicious anemia in Boston.

Dogs that had been bled were not similar to humans with pernicious anemia. The reasons for the anemia were different, but Minot and Murphy were intrigued and impressed by Whipple's findings. They decided to use these results in their own work. In 1926, Minot and Murphy found that if a person ill with pernicious anemia could eat half a pound of fresh or lightly cooked liver every day, he or she would recover. The researchers did not know which substance in liver treated the anemia in the humans and the dogs. It turns out that liver cures anemia in bled dogs and pernicious anemia in humans in different ways. We now know that Whipple's dogs improved because of the iron in the liver. Iron was not the substance that cured pernicious anemia because pernicious anemia is not due to iron deficiency or to any dietary deficiency, but the work of Minot and Murphy made it clear that pernicious anemia, whatever its cause, could be treated by diet. Whipple, Minot, and Murphy received the Nobel Prize in Physiology, or Medicine, in 1934 for their discovery that liver treated pernicious anemia.

Large quantities of liver remained the treatment for patients with pernicious anemia, but this treatment was difficult to tolerate. We have an account of this from an unexpected source. In a biography of Linus Pauling, the author describes the illness of Pauling's mother: "She began suffering from a general weakness that was later diagnosed as pernicious anemia, a ruinous, energy-sapping blood disorder . . . Her doctor did all he could, prescribing long periods of rest and a diet rich in red meats designed to build the blood. The children would later remember the copious amounts of liver she ate, and 'cannibal sandwiches' made of raw beef scrapings and blood on bread. . . ."[3] Some have wondered whether the illness of Pauling's mother was one of the reasons that he became interested later in his professional life in medicine.

A Meat Chopper, a Yellow Bowl, and a Stomach Tube

William Bosworth Castle (1897–1990) and his colleagues at the Thorndike Memorial Laboratory at Boston City Hospital investigated the liver cure. They knew that patients with pernicious anemia had shrunken stomachs and produced stomach juice with less acid than did healthy people. Replacement of an ill person's stomach juices with those of a well person was ineffective in treating the illness. Castle put this finding together with the finding of Minot and Murphy that large amounts of liver cured pernicious anemia and concluded that there must be two factors present to prevent pernicious anemia: one present in healthy stomach juice, which he called the *intrinsic factor*, and one present in some foods, which he called the *extrinsic factor*. He suspected an interaction between these two factors. Large amounts of *extrinsic factor* found in liver were able to compensate for the ill person's lack of *intrinsic factor*. Castle performed a series of experiments to demonstrate the existence of these two factors and the relationship between them:

> Thus Castle began a therapeutic trial that required him to consume 300 g of rare hamburg steak daily for 10 days, extract his own stomach contents after an hour, allow this to incubate for a few hours until liquefied, and then administer the mixture to an anemic patient through a flexible stomach tube of small caliber . . . Castle's laboratory equipment for observations that turned out to have far-reaching consequences was by today's standards deceptively simple: a meat chopper, a yellow bowl, a 6-inch fine wire mesh strainer, a Rehfuss stomach tube, liquid pH indicators, beakers, a microscope, and stains for blood films and reticulocytes. The indispensable instrument of Castle's scientific procedure was, of course, the pernicious anemia patient under his immediate, concerned and grateful care. . . .[4]

The timing was important. In other experiments, Castle had already shown that stomach juice, when given separately from the hamburg steak, had no effect. The stomach juice and steak had to be present together. Something had to happen *between* the factor in the stomach juice and the factor in the hamburg steak. The experiment described above worked well. The bone marrow of the patients began to make red blood cells. This work showed, in a compelling manner, a very clear connection between the stomach and the bone marrow.

The writer of this account pays graceful tribute to Castle's ill patients, which is quite unusual in the history of medicine. The patient recognized that Castle was concerned for his or her welfare, yet the patient did not realize just how closely involved Castle was. The patients were not told the origin of this substance in the flexible stomach tube. One can imagine the hesitation that an ill patient (or anyone) would have in consuming his or her doctor's regurgitated meal. It is difficult to know how to classify this experiment. In a sense, it was self-experimentation, similar to what was done by Goldberger, in that Castle inflicted discomfort on himself while performing a medical experiment. However, Castle administered the results of his experiment to ill patients. Goldberger experimented on himself and *fully informed* healthy volunteers to see whether he could *cause* illness. Castle experimented on himself and then on *uninformed* ill patients, trying to *treat* the illness. Castle's experiment could not have been done today because of the element of deception. This important experiment was not used in actual practice. Castle and others were eventually able to prepare concentrated extracts of liver that patients found less odious to eat. They also discovered that injections of this extract worked better than giving it by mouth.

It took another twenty years of work to define the nature of the substance in hamburg steak and liver that cured the anemia—and why it worked better by injection. This substance, Castle's extrinsic factor, turned out to be cobalamin, Vitamin B12. The gastric factor, a large protein, was the intrinsic factor as it continues to be known today. In another odd coincidence, Castle was the person who first mentioned to Linus Pauling that red blood cells were "twisted" in patients with sickle-cell anemia. This conversation led Pauling to discover the cause of that illness and is described at greater length in the Vitamin C chapter.

Explanation for Castle's Success

Castle's experiment worked in this way. He ate the hamburg steak, and his stomach acid separated the Vitamin B12 from accompanying proteins. Castle's regurgitated stomach contents included freed Vitamin B12 but also another important molecule, intrinsic factor. His intrinsic factor bound to the Vitamin B12 to form a stable compound. When Castle's stomach contents were administered to the anemic patient, the anemic patient was then able to absorb the Vitamin B12-intrinsic factor compound.

Vitamin B12 Absorption and Vitamin B12 Deficiency Anemias

There must be a supply of Vitamin B12 in the diet; this usually comes from meat. Many people consume meat-free or meat-poor diets because of choice or poverty. These people may develop Vitamin B12 dietary or nutritional deficiency anemias.

Vitamin B12 deficiency is not always a nutritional deficiency disorder. Even if the diet contains adequate Vitamin B12, the vitamin still has to be absorbed, which takes many steps. There are several opportunities for something to go awry in the lengthy process of Vitamin B12 absorption. Vitamin B12 in food is tightly bound to proteins and must be freed from these proteins by saliva enzymes and acid found in stomach juices. The freed vitamin is then rebound to the large stomach protein, intrinsic factor. This stable complex travels the length of the small intestine, and it is finally absorbed in the last part of the small intestine.

The vitamin may be difficult to digest if there is not enough stomach acid to separate the Vitamin B12 from other proteins. This is often the case in older people. If there are any diseases or problems with the stomach or bowel, Vitamin B12 anemia can result. The classic though rare cause of low Vitamin B12 is pernicious anemia. Pernicious anemia is an autoimmune illness in which there are destructive antibodies both to the cells, which make the intrinsic factor, and to the intrinsic factor itself.

Purifying the Anti-Anemia Factor

Scientists knew that Castle's extrinsic factor in the liver was the anti-anemia factor. The liver is the center of much of the body's metabolism and makes bile, cholesterol, and albumin, among many other substances, and detoxifies harmful substances. The liver stores sugar and a number of vitamins. Finding the one molecule that was the extrinsic factor in the middle of this complex organ was a daunting task.

Because the marketing opportunities were significant, chemists at pharmaceutical companies competed to find the factor. In 1948, Karl Folkers from Merck Laboratories in the United States isolated a substance from liver as the pure anti-anemia factor. At the same time, in England, Dr. E. Lester Smith and his research group at the pharmaceutical company Glaxo reported that they had found the vitamin. Merck and Alexander Todd in Cambridge, England, both showed that the newly named Vitamin B12 contained cobalt, a metal. This was a surprise because this element appears nowhere else in the human body, but they were still not sure of the actual composition of the vitamin. The Glaxo group gave the small, deep-red, needle-like crystals to Dorothy Crowfoot Hodgkin and her Oxford X-ray crystallography group in England so that they could help them to work out the details of the vitamin. X-ray crystallography is a technique used by chemists to establish three-dimensional structures of molecules. Many thought that this would be an impossible task because cobalamin was so large and complicated.

Dorothy Crowfoot Hodgkin, Collaboration, and Cobalamin Crystals: "Pure Brain Work—and Mosaics All Over Again . . ."

Dorothy Crowfoot Hodgkin (1910–1994) was born in Cairo to a highly educated English family. Her father was a civil servant in the British administration of Egypt and an amateur archaeologist. Her mother, also interested in archaeology, was an expert in weaving. As a schoolgirl, Dorothy became interested in chemistry, crystals, and the more abstract subject of structure and patterns. When she was fifteen, her mother gave her copies of lectures written by Sir William Bragg, a Nobel Prize winner in physics, about the use of X-rays to study materials. Mother and daughter read these lectures together. Hodgkin wrote about this interest that she shared with her mother:

> [My mother] was particularly fascinated by the discovery of the arrangements in different materials, potsherds and cotton and linen fibres, in which she was interested for archaeological reasons. I was fascinated by the way this knowledge was acquired—by passing X-rays through crystals and studying the diffraction effects produced by the atoms on X-rays. I began to see X-ray diffraction as a means to exploring many of the questions raised but left unanswered by school chemistry—the structure of solids and of biological materials.[5]

She joined her parents on a dig in Jordan and wrote about the fifth- and sixth-century mosaics: "The pattern in the nave was of linked octagons, and there were small panels, square or diamond-shaped, generally with decorative motifs between them . . . I began to think of the restraints imposed by two-dimensional order in a plane."[6] Hodgkin left the excavations of the past and began to explore the structures of the natural world. She studied chemistry at Oxford University from 1928 to 1932 and became more interested in crystallography. In a letter written to her parents, she agonized about the difficulties she would be facing:

> . . . I'm feeling quite appalled at the prospect. There will be such a fearful lot of work—and mathematics—involved. And I was just beginning to rejoice so much in the idea of a nice quiet organic research that would involve no brain whatever. As it is, it will be practically pure brain work—and mosaics all over again . . . It is one thing to appreciate the structures that other people have worked out for crystals—and quite another to be able to work them out for yourself. The first requires the same faculties I apply to mosaics—the second requires pure mathematics. It is quite dreadful to think about it . . . Of course, if I can really do it it will be rather priceless . . .[7]

Hodgkin had the qualities needed to be a good X-ray crystallographer. She understood chemistry well, saw structures in a three-dimensional way, and was ready to take on a "fearful lot of work." Using the cumbersome and tedious X-ray techniques of the day, Hodgkin and her group determined an actual chemical formula for several large biological molecules with the aid of X-ray diffraction. In their long years of work with Vitamin B12, they were the first to determine the structure of a metalloenzyme, a protein containing a metal within its structure. Hodgkin and her group discovered other unexpected chemical features, such as a strange ring of nitrogens and carbons surrounding the cobalt. They determined the correct structures of other important biological molecules, including penicillin and insulin.

X-RAY CRYSTALLOGRAPHY: A WAY OF "SEEING" PROTEIN MOLECULES

We see objects because rays of visible light bounce off, or are diffracted by, the object, and then are focused through the lens of our eyes. This depends on two factors:

- the object being larger than rays of visible light.
- the ability of visible light rays to be focused through a lens.

Visible light is electromagnetic radiation, with wavelengths of 400–700 nm. A molecule is much smaller than this wavelength, so radiation with a far smaller wavelength is used to "see" molecules. The wavelength of the radiation used in X-ray crystallography is about .01–10 nm. Unlike visible light, it cannot be focused through a lens.

   To obtain images of protein molecules, protein crystals must be formed. Crystals of proteins contain molecules in highly ordered three-dimensional arrays. It is a delicate process to find the right solution in which to dissolve the protein and the right speed at which then to evaporate the water so that crystals form. Once a crystal is formed, the crystallographer uses an X-ray source to bombard the crystal with beams of radiation. The crystal is rotated, and multiple diffraction patterns are collected. An X-ray film (or the equivalent) detects the diffracted X-rays. The pattern produced is complex, does not bear a simple relationship to the crystal, and must be interpreted with the aid of intuition and complex data analysis.

Pharmaceutical companies, such as Glaxo and Merck, needed to know the structure of the vitamin before they could manufacture it. Glaxo supported Hodgkin's work with Vitamin B12. Merck supported other crystallographers. For Hodgkin and her collaborators, the search was quite different than it was for the companies. The scientists were competing with each other for the academic recognition, but also for the sheer enjoyment of deciphering molecular structure. Hodgkin was not concerned about Glaxo's share of the cobalamin market. She was friendly with her competitors. In an interview, she explained her collaboration with the chemists at Merck, "We were formally supposed to be rivals. But after a time, when we were dreadfully bogged down, we went into collusion. I think we were regarded as wholly unreliable by the firms to which we were attached, and we ended up publishing jointly."[8] Sheer enjoyment had trumped commercial competition.

Hodgkin was one of the first crystallographers to work with computers. The computers made the calculations easier, but they were still time-consuming. Kenneth Trueblood (1920–1998), a California scientist, was visiting Oxford in 1953 and worked with Hodgkin. He had access to one of the world's fastest and most complex computers at the time. Trueblood returned to Los Angeles, and with one his students, Dick Prosen, entered Hodgkin's crystallographic data into the American computer. Trueblood and Prosen worked at night, because that was when the computers were available. Trueblood also taught during the day. He described their work:

> What it involved was sitting at a card punch typewriter with a stack of IBM cards in a machine, and you hope you get all the numbers in the right places. And first you type up the intensity data, 3000 pieces of data each with a triple of indices, so you type 7 4 10 and then 193, and then 7 4 11 and 20, and then 7 4 12 37 and so on. And then you print them out and proofread them and correct your errors. Then you take another set of punched cards and you put in the positions of each of the atoms that they've so far identified . . . Dick Prosen and I worked 12 hours at a stretch, all night. It [the computer] increased the speed at which you could do this by a factor of maybe 100, so we could do in one night what would have taken three or four months.[9]

With the help of this Californian nocturnal toil, and also the work of many other colleagues in England, Hodgkin finally established the structure of Vitamin B12 in 1955. It had taken the team eight years. In 1964 the Nobel Prize in Chemistry was awarded to Hodgkin for her work with cobalamin.

Hodgkin was generous and enthusiastic in work with scientists in less developed countries. She traveled to the Soviet Union, China, and India and helped many crystallographers in these countries. She also became, as had Linus Pauling, interested in left-wing causes and pacifism.

Like Pauling, she was not trusted by her own government because of these interests and her frequent trips abroad. However, one of her students was the far-from-left-wing Margaret Thatcher. As might have been predicted by

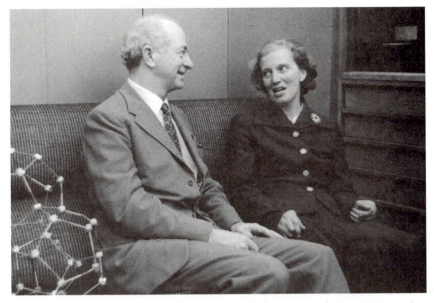

Linus Pauling (1901–1994) and Dorothy Hodgkin (1910–1994) shared interests in crystallography and politics. Both at times were restricted from traveling by their respective governments. Note the molecular model beside Pauling, and Hodgkin's hands, crippled by rheumatoid arthritis, which did not hinder her from her work with crystals. This was taken in 1957. Courtesy Ava Helen and Linus Pauling Papers, Oregon State University Libraries Special Collections.

Hodgkin's ability to cooperate with her competitor from Merck, she was able to stay on good terms with the English Prime Minister, despite their political differences. In addition to the Nobel Prize, Hodgkin won a Lenin Peace Prize in 1987 in recognition for her work in easing tensions between the east and the west during the cold war.

Cobalamin, Methane, Mud, and Sludge: Discoveries from the San Francisco Bay

Cobalamin is synthesized by small microorganisms associated with fermentation, a process of decomposition in which various substances are broken down. Fermentation is sometimes carried out by anaerobic microorganisms in the absence of air or oxygen. Anaerobic fermentation produces methane, also known as marsh gas, because it is so often produced in the muck of ponds and marshes. Dr. Thressa Stadtman, a scientist at the National Institutes of Health, investigated the activities of bacteria that live in oxygen-free or anaerobic environments. She showed that methane-producing, anaerobic bacteria from the mud of San Francisco Bay synthesized Vitamin B12 compounds. Later work with Vitamin B12 compounds was made easier by the finding that the final steps in fermentation of sludge in sewage plants are carried out by anaerobic bacteria, which produce methane—and Vitamin B compounds.

Another place where both methane and cobalamin are produced is the rumen of the cow. The rumen is a large, complicated fermentation vat containing microbes that ferment the cellulose in cereals and grains. (This is why cows can grow on grass, and we cannot.) The cow takes in some cobalt from the grasses. Anaerobic bacteria in the rumen form many compounds including several B vitamins. Cows eructate ("burp") huge quantities of methane. The B vitamins made by the microorganisms are absorbed into the animal tissue. The consumption of animal products, such as beef or liver, is our main source of cobalamin.

METHANE

Methane is a simple molecule made of one carbon atom and four hydrogens. It is the main component of natural gas and is a widely used energy source. It is also a greenhouse gas that contributes to global warming. It is produced by the compression of organic matter deep in the earth or by anaerobic fermentation. Without anaerobic fermentation and the production of methane, we would be buried under organic matter, such as sewage and dead plant matter, which would not decay, and we would be without Vitamin B12.

Synthesis of Cobalamin: 100 Researchers and 100 Reactions

The structure of cobalamin was difficult to determine, and the vitamin was also difficult to reproduce in the laboratory. Vitamin B12 is the largest and most complicated vitamin, consisting of 181 atoms. Vitamin C, in comparison, contains only twenty atoms. Robert Burns Woodward (1917–1979) had been awarded a Nobel Prize for Chemistry in 1965 for his synthesis of complex organic molecules. In collaboration with Albert Eschenmoser (1925–), a renowned chemist from Zurich, and, over a decade, with about one hundred other coworkers, Woodward synthesized cobalamin by a sequence of more than one hundred reactions. They completed this task in 1971. From isolation to synthesis took twenty-three years. Folate, in comparison, was isolated and synthesized in a mere three years.

Putting the Fruit Bat at Risk

Only a few species of bacteria living in sewage, mud, and the rumens of some animals are able to make this complicated molecule. Ruminants have bacteria in their rumens, which synthesize the cobalamin, which is then absorbed into the animal tissue. Most humans get Vitamin B12 by eating meat from these animals. Because Vitamin B12 is not found in plants, vegetarians are at risk of Vitamin B12 deficiency. Many people eat little meat, through poverty, lack of availability, or choice, yet few of these people suffer from Vitamin B12 deficiency. How is that? It has long been suspected that perhaps

Vitamin B12 is available through microbial contamination of fruits and vegetables. This theory has been supported by some clever work with bats.

The small Egyptian fruit bat (*Rousettus aegyptiacus*) is just like a human: it needs Vitamin B12 but cannot make it. The Egyptian fruit bat is frugivorous, meaning that it only eats fruit. Scientists in South America studied captive fruit bats. They also wondered how these mammals survived without B12. They found that if the captive is supplied only with washed and peeled fruit, the bat develops signs of Vitamin B12 deficiency.[10] The lesson is that vigorously washing fruit in some situations might lead to Vitamin B12 deficiency. Cow manure contains Vitamin B12, and perhaps some people who eat no meat obtain their vitamin from eating vegetables that are contaminated by fertilizer containing dung.

SYNTHESIS OF COMPLICATED MOLECULES BY BACTERIA

Streptomyces griseus, a soil microbe, was found in a clump of dirt taken from the throat of a sick chicken. This microbe makes streptomycin, the first medication useful in the therapy of tuberculosis. Folkers at Merck, who had found cobalamin in the liver, showed that *Streptomyces* also makes Vitamin B12. Other humble anaerobic bacteria living in sludge and rumens also synthesize this vitamin. Microorganisms have been doing this for billions of years.

Consequences of Vitamin B12 Deficiency: Megaloblastic Madness

Vitamin B12 deficiency, like folate deficiency, causes a macrocytic anemia. There are medical problems associated with Vitamin B12 deficiency that do not occur in folate deficiency. The Vitamin B12-deficient person may have a sore tongue, difficulty walking, confusion, and unpleasant feelings in his or her hands and feet, described as tingling or "pins and needles." Bowel and bladder control can be disturbed. These symptoms are constant, progressive, and distressing. In the past, often as part of pernicious anemia, severe psychiatric problems developed. A young British physician in 1960 described some typical cases:

- A forty-eight-year-old woman was referred to the outpatient department because of sleeplessness, giddiness, and a feeling as if she was walking on air. She was unable to hold things in her right arm because of numbness and a feeling of "pins-and-needles." Later, she was admitted to the hospital because of depression and suicidal thoughts. A sister had died about twenty-five years earlier from anemia while still in her twenties.
- A thirty-four-year-old woman developed a sore tongue and a sensation of electricity in her arms and legs. She thought that she smelled offensively, and told her children not to eat the food she had prepared. She became more depressed and tried to drown herself.
- A forty-four-year-old woman was diagnosed with pernicious anemia but could not eat the prescribed amount of liver. Twenty years later, she was described as "mentally strange and talking nonsense" and was admitted to a hospital.[11]

In all of the cases listed above, the patients improved once given Vitamin B12. The physician who described these cases coined the term *megaloblastic madness.* Physicians reported that neurological symptoms of patients with pernicious anemia worsened when given folate.[12] It is now part of routine medical practice to check Vitamin B12 levels in patients with complaints of sore tongue, pain or numbness in their limbs, or psychiatric problems, such as confusion or depression.

SUMMARY

Bone marrow makes millions of red blood cells every minute and depends on folate and cobalamin to do this. These two vitamins are needed for the synthesis, repair, and normal functioning of deoxyribonucleic acid required for the production and maintenance of new red cells. Folate was discovered in foods that few people eat—liver, Marmite, and spinach. Now, we know that folate is found in a number of vegetables and fruit. Folate fortification in the United States, beginning in 1998, has increased folic acid blood levels. The consequences of this are still being studied.

Lucy Wills and Dorothy Hodgkin were two young women from privileged English families who each had a penchant for travel and adventure. Wills was one of the first researchers to show the close connection between stomach and bone marrow, while working in the laboratories of Bombay with rats and monkeys. Hodgkin, working in the more famous laboratories of Oxford, only a few decades later, worked with more rarefied material—crystals and computers. Their work, along with that of researchers who bled dogs and treated patients with their own stomach juices, proved that a varied diet is essential for healthy blood and, as shown in later work, for healthy babies and strong nervous systems.

5

SAILORS, SCURVY, THE GUINEA PIG, AND THE NOBEL PRIZE: VITAMIN C (ASCORBIC ACID), THE ANTI-SCURVY VITAMIN

OVERVIEW

Vitamin C, or ascorbic acid, is the best known and simplest of all of the vitamins. Deficiency of this small molecule leads to the terrible illness scurvy, which causes fatigue, rashes, and swollen and bleeding gums. Ascorbic acid means "without scurvy."

The history of scurvy is full of adventure and paradox. It involves journeys around the world, to the South Pacific, and to the frozen reaches of the Arctic. French sailors trapped in the frozen St. Lawrence River in Quebec and English sailors tacking across the Mediterranean and the English Channel suffered from scurvy. The cure for scurvy was often found and often forgotten. Dr. James Lind, the man who most clearly showed that oranges and lemons treated scurvy and, in so doing, performed the first controlled trial in medicine, was never quite sure that he was correct. By the end of his life, he had given up his interest in citrus fruits for an older interest—sweat. The English navy—many decades after Lind's work—insisted that all sailors drink lime or lemon juice, thus leading to the name of "limey" for the British. Scurvy disappeared from the navy but continued to cause anguish in the Arctic, the Crimea, and the children of the wealthy.

Much useful laboratory work was done by two Nobel Prize–winning scientists. Albert Szent-Györgyi, a colorful Hungarian count, discovered the structure of Vitamin C in red pepper fields. Linus Pauling, one of the most respected and influential scientists of our time, made the vitamin famous, yet his work in this area is not taken seriously by the medical establishment. He was monitored closely by the Federal Bureau of Investigation (FBI) for over two decades because of his work in the peace movement.

Scurvy and the Age of Discovery

Scurvy has been recognized for many centuries, but it is particularly associated with long sea voyages of the 1500s to 1800s. Scurvy is a disease of nautical progress and adventure. When boats were small and could not travel far from shore, sailors did not develop scurvy. It was only as boats became bigger and navigation became more skillful that long voyages could be undertaken, and the conditions for scurvy could develop.

During the Age of Discovery, from the early fifteenth century through the early seventeenth century, European ships sailed around the world. They were searching for gold, silver, and spices and new trading routes and partners. The sagas of the great European adventurers usually concentrate on the exotic sites to which they traveled and the bravery and adroit navigation of the captains and their sailors. The tales rarely focus on the enormous loss of life that was a feature of these trips and that was usually caused by scurvy. As we saw with the conquistadors in Central and South America, the medical and nutritional consequences of adventure are overlooked.

In 1498, Vasco da Gama (1460–1524) of Portugal sailed east. He rounded the Cape of Good Hope at the southern tip of Africa and sailed up the east coast of Africa to what is now Mombasa, Kenya. His sailors were saved from scurvy by African traders who supplied them with oranges and lemons. He traveled on across the Indian Ocean and reached Calicut. After four months, he returned to Portugal. The trip was a success in that he was the first man to sail from Europe to India. It was a failure in that many sailors, including his own brother, died from scurvy on the return trip. Another Portuguese explorer, Ferdinand Magellan (1480–1521), was sent by Spain on a westward trip to find spices. He left Spain in 1519 with five ships. He sailed through the straits that separate the southern tip of South America and Tierra del Fuego, subsequently named the Straits of Magellan, to the Spice Islands in the Pacific Ocean, where he picked up cloves and cinnamon. After fifteen weeks at sea, many of the sailors suffered terribly from scurvy. In his journals, Magellan described the illness:

> Wednesday, the twenty-eighth of November, 1520, we came forth out of the said strait, and entered into the Pacific sea, where we remained three months and twenty days without taking in provisions or other refreshments, and we only ate old biscuit reduced to powder, and full of grubs, and stinking from the dirt which the rats had made on it when eating the good biscuit . . . the upper and lower gums of most of our men grew so much that they could not eat and in this way so many suffered. . . .[1]

Magellan died in a battle at the Philippines. Only one ship returned to Seville in 1522. Magellan led the first successful trip around the world, but he and 252 of his original 270 sailors did not return home. Many of the deaths were due to scurvy.

Admiral George Anson (1697–1762) circumnavigated the world during a war between England and Spain. In 1740 Anson and a small armada left England and chased after the Spanish fleet across the oceans of the world. After three years of pursuit, near misses, storms at sea, navigational mishaps, and sea fights, Anson was left with only one small ship. Even so, he captured a Spanish treasure galleon, the immensely rich *Nuestra Señora de Covadonga*, containing gold from Mexico. He sold her cargo to the Chinese and returned home to England in 1744 a rich man. Of nineteen hundred sailors, fourteen hundred died. Most of the deaths were caused by scurvy. The enemy in this story was never the Spanish—it was scurvy. Vitamin C deficiency, not Spanish swords or gunfire, killed Anson's English seamen. They would have fared better if *Nuestra Señora de Covadonga* had been full of sauerkraut and lemons rather than pieces of gold. Anson was much lauded in England for his perseverance and doughty spirit. He was an English swashbuckling hero. (To the Spanish, he was a pirate.) Anson's adventures and exploits led to his ascendancy in the admiralty. Because of this, he was able to be helpful to one of our later heroes—James Lind.

Da Gama, Magellan, and Anson were brilliant sea captains, but their trips were achieved at the cost of the deaths of most of their crews. Why did so many sailors die from scurvy on these voyages? In Magellan's description of the illness, a connection between the poor food and the disease jumps out at the modern reader. Their food consisted of salted meat, weevily biscuit, and no fresh fruits or vegetables. The ships had poor food for several reasons. The ships were teeming with sailors, at least at the outset of the voyages. Because so many sailors died, far more sailors than were actually needed were recruited at the beginning of voyages. The ships were also loaded with heavy sails, rigging, cargo, guns, and ammunition, all of which occupied much space. Therefore, there was little room for food. There was no refrigeration and no airtight storage. Salted meat and biscuits were compact, cheap, and able to withstand months or years of storage at sea. The choice of these foods was sensible given these circumstances and what was known then about nutrition—nothing.

Cures for Scurvy

Scurvy was an illness with an easy-to-discover cure. One of the earliest and most dramatic "discoveries" of the cure for scurvy took place in French Canada. Jacques Cartier had landed in Quebec in the winter of 1535–1536. The winter was severe, and his three ships were frozen in the Saint Lawrence River. Most of the men became ill with scurvy. Cartier saw that the Native Americans of Stadacona also became ill and had a cure. The Indians gave their cure to Cartier:

> In the month of December we received warning that the pestilence had broken out among the people of Stadacona to such an extent, that already, by their own confession, more than fifty persons were dead. Upon this we forbade them to come either to the fort or about us. But notwithstanding we had driven them away, the sickness broke out among us accompanied by most marvelous and extraordinary symptoms; for some lost all their strength, their legs became swollen and inflamed, while the sinews contracted and turned as black as coal. In other

cases the legs were found blotched with purple coloured blood. Then the disease would mount to the hips, thighs, shoulders, arms and neck. And all had their mouths so tainted, that the gums rotted away down to the roots of the teeth, which nearly all fell out . . . We were also in great dread of the people of the country, lest they should become aware of our plight and helplessness . . . From the middle of November 1535 until Saturday the fifteenth of April 1536, we lay frozen up in the ice, which was more than two fathoms in thickness, while on shore there were more than 4 ft. of snow . . . One day our Captain . . . caught sight of a band of Indians approaching from Stadacona, and among them was Dom Agaya whom he had seen ten or twelve days previous to this, extremely ill with the very disease his own men were suffering from . . . when the Indians had come near the fort, the Captain inquired of him (Dom Agaya), what had cured him of his sickness. Dom Agaya replied that he had been healed by the juice of the leaves of a tree and the dregs of these, and that this was the only way to cure the sickness . . . They showed us how to grind the bark and the leaves and to boil the whole in water . . . The Captain at once ordered a drink to be prepared . . . As soon as they had drunk it, they felt better which must be ascribed to miraculous causes; for after drinking it two or three times, they recovered health and strength and were cured of all the diseases they ever had. . . .[2]

This story illustrates the complex relationship between the Europeans and the native Indians. The French were afraid of "catching" scurvy from the Indians and then were afraid of being attacked by them. In fact, the Indians behaved charitably toward the French. (As was described in the chapter about Vitamin B3, the native Indians would also be helpful to the English pilgrims a century later.) Cartier called Dom Agaya's cure miraculous and noted that all of their diseases were cured. This is a testament to the severity of the illness and the rapidity with which Vitamin C could cure it. Cartier knew that the "miracle" was an infusion of bark and leaves. He did not understand that this infusion was replacing a deficiency in the diet of his men. The actual plant used by Dom Agaya and his band remains unknown. Scholars have suggested spruce, pine, or sassafras. Cartier seems not to have told other explorers about it, and scurvy remained problematic among the early European settlers of North America.

Sailors from all parts of the world had noticed the connection between citrus fruit or fresh vegetables and the improved health of their sailors. For example, Sir Richard Hawkins (1562–1622) sailed to the South Seas in 1593. He described scurvy and the relief that his sailors found from eating citrus fruit, yet he never took the next step of including citrus fruit in his own supplies or suggesting citrus fruit to others. In 1601, Sir John Lancaster of the East India Company suggested that citrus fruit be supplied to all sailors, thinking that this would somehow counter the ill effects of the diet of salt meat. John Woodall (1556–1643), the assistant surgeon of the East India Company, suggested that scurvy resulted from an inadequate diet and recommended fresh food as a treatment. If fresh food was not available, he recommended that oranges, lemons, limes, tamarinds (a tropical fruit), or oil of vitriol (sulfuric acid) be used. Woodall and others believed that it was the acidity of these substances that was helpful.

In 1734, Dr. Johannes Bachstrom (1688–1742), a Dutch physician, coined the word "anti-scorbutic," meaning "without scurvy" and applied it to fresh vegetables. He was the first person to suggest that scurvy could be a deficiency disease. He recommended that everyone should eat more fresh vegetables. This excellent advice went unheeded by most. One remarkable scholar who did pay attention was an Italian physician and Freemason. Antonio Cocchi (1695–1758) was Professor of Medicine at Pisa. He was a vegetarian who believed that vegetables were acidic and therefore easy to digest. Meat in contrast was oily and caused "glutinous blockages." Cocchi relied in part on Pythagoras (ca. 575 to 495 BCE), an earlier vegetarian, who, he believed, had an enlightened and scientific understanding of diet. Pythagoras, an ancient Greek, was an important man to have on one's side. In the sixteenth century, there had been a resurgence of interest in the wisdom of ancient Greece. The educated European believed that the finest thinking of the world had occurred in the minds of the inhabitants of ancient Greece. This admiration could be detrimental to the progress of medicine, as we shall see when we review some of the theories as to the causes of scurvy.

Cocchi visited England, joined the Freemasons, returned to Italy, and established the first Masonic lodge in Florence. Cocchi wrote a history of Freemasonry and connected it with Pythagorean philosophy, the ancient Egyptians, Galileo's discovery of the Earth rotating around the Sun, and vegetarianism. He read Bachstrom. Cocchi's mind was fertile soil for Bachstrom's thesis because of his own vegetarianism. Cocchi wrote that scurvy was caused by not eating vegetables. Bachstrom and Cocchi were correct. Their suggestions that people eat more fresh vegetables made no impact on the medical or government bodies of the day. Even with the support of Pythagoras, they were ignored.

Why was this? The cause of scurvy, obvious to us, was obscured by other problems associated with scurvy. Those who developed scurvy were often living in difficult conditions, and it was difficult to separate out what was relevant to the scurvy and what was just making the scurvy even more miserable. Many had drawn conclusions from a series of observations. Others had come to conclusions based on their understanding of Greek medical theories. Much of the theorizing was based on the ancient supposition that there are four bodily fluids or humors: yellow bile, blood, phlegm, and black bile. This system was propagated by Hippocrates (ca. 460 BCE–ca. 370 BCE) and Galen of Pergamum (130–201). Each humor was associated with two of the four fundamental qualities; hot, cold, wet, and dry; and one of four elements: air, fire, earth, or water. Blood was associated with warmth, moisture, and air. Diseases developed if there was an excess, deterioration, or curdling of any of the humors. Sweating or perspiring was an important way of balancing the humors and ridding the body of poisons.

Proposed Causes of Scurvy Based on Observations

Fatigue, depression, homesickness, contagion, seawater, damp air, copper pans, tobacco, hot climate, cold climate, rats, heredity, contagion, fresh fruit, too much exercise, too little exercise, sea air, salted meat, poor morals, and filth.

These elusive substances caused all illnesses. Since the humors couldn't actually be measured, it was possible for scholars to generate theories that could never be disproved. Academicians were often determined to follow the teachings of the ancients and frequently resorted to machinations of logic to reach their conclusions. Theories were produced aplenty. They were complex and irrelevant to the actual diseases.

Proposed Causes of Scurvy Based on Theories

Alkalinity, acidity, too much fixed air, too little fixed air, putrefaction, too much black bile, corruption of the humors, and blocked perspiration.

Little was understood then about digestion. The idea that we needed to eat a variety of foods was not obvious. The observations of Cartier and others did not fit the current humoral theories, so they were ignored by the medical establishment. Those who had suggested fresh food or citrus fruits, such as Hawkins, Lancaster, and Woodall, did not have a theory that made their suggestions appealing. Bachstrom's concept of dietary deficiency did not fit easily into humorism. Cocchi's reliance on Pythagoras in his attempt to convince people to eat more fresh vegetables was no match for the academicians who believed in Galen's humors.

Dr. James Lind and His Trial

The English navy became more concerned about scurvy in the 1700s, when the navy became an integral part of the defense of England against France and Spain, and the health of the English seaman became a matter of national importance. Dr. James Lind (1716–1794), the most famous person in the history of scurvy and Vitamin C, was an English naval physician who proved that citrus fruits cured scurvy. Despite his definitive experiment on board the *HMS Salisbury*, he never embraced his own findings.

Lind was born in Edinburgh and became a surgeon's mate in the English navy in 1739. He served in the Mediterranean, off the coast of West Africa, and in the West Indies. During these trips, he saw many cases of scurvy. Eventually, he became a naval surgeon, which was then a few steps below the position of doctor. In 1747, Lind was serving as naval surgeon on the *HMS Salisbury*. Lind did not have strong beliefs about the correct way to treat scurvy, but he did want to know how to prevent or treat it, so he decided to find out for himself the best way of doing this.

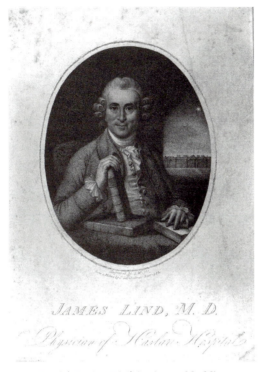

James Lind (1716–1794) is pictured holding
Treatise of the Scurvy. The navy hospital, Haslar, is
in the background. Wellcome Library, London.

Large ships were a good "laboratory" for experiments because sailors on these ships were a "captive" group. The situation was somewhat similar to that of the Javanese road builders or prisoners in Governor Brewer's Mississippi Rankin Farm reviewed in earlier chapters. Lind took twelve sailors ill with scurvy and divided them into six pairs. He treated each pair with one of six treatments, each of which had been described as an effective cure for scurvy. The sailors stayed in the sick bay of the *Salisbury* during the trial and were fed the same diet, consisting of gruel for breakfast, mutton broth and pudding for lunch, and barley with sage for supper.

The men eating the citrus fruit became well within six days and actually helped to care for the other ill men. The other men remained ill. This was a landmark result. Lind had advanced medical science in two important ways. First, he had "controlled" the study by making sure that all of the subjects were similar and exposed to the same conditions; only the treatment was different. Thus, it was clear that whichever pair of sailors did best, it could only

---

THE TREATMENTS IN LIND'S TRIAL

1. One quart of cider
2. Twenty-five drops of elixir of vitriol (sulfuric acid) three times a day
3. Two spoonfuls of vinegar three times a day
4. Half a pint of seawater
5. Two oranges and one lemon for six days, after which the supply was exhausted
6. An "electuary" (a pasty mix of medicinal substances) the size of a nutmeg, made up of garlic, mustard seed, balsam of Peru, dried radish root, and gum myrrh (a resin), along with barley water treated with tamarinds and cremor tartor (a leftover substance from winemaking)

---

be caused by the difference in their treatments. This was one of the first controlled clinical trials in medicine. Second, he demonstrated that the cure for scurvy was citrus fruit.

In 1748, Lind retired from the navy and wrote *Treatise on the Scurvy*, in which he reviewed the previous literature and described his own powerful and convincing trial. He published his four-hundred-page treatise in 1753. Famously—nothing happened. The English authorities ignored this book, to much scorn and derision of later critics. Why did the publication of this book cause so little stir? Lind had reviewed the literature about scurvy and produced a massive tome that was impossible to read. He had surveyed the mystifying muddle of beliefs about humors, putrefaction, fermentation, acidity, and fixed air. He had been unable to bring any clarity to this jumble. His scholarly activity had led to a complex and turgid book.

He described his experiment in five paragraphs, which were hidden among descriptions of impressions of others and humors. Lind did not, out of modesty or uncertainty, highlight his own simple and convincing trial. By the time he finished his treatise, it is as though he was exhausted and lost. Moreover, he did not make any clear recommendations. Lind suggested hesitantly and with much qualification that the navy use "rob," a heated and condensed form of citrus juice, to treat scurvy. As we shall see later, Lind was correct in being lukewarm about this suggestion. Scientists are sometimes accused of improving their results or making too much of them. If there is any scientist innocent of this, it must be James Lind. One task of any researcher is to doubt his or her own findings and to look for alternative explanations. If there is any researcher who doubted, it must be James Lind.

In 1758, Anson, the sea pirate–circumnavigator, appointed Lind, by then a more prestigious physician, to be in charge of the large naval hospital at Haslar, Portsmouth. Lind continued to work with patients ill with scurvy. Lind produced a third edition of the *Treatise* in 1772, in which he reported on his experience at Haslar. During these years, he had supervised the care of thousands of patients with scurvy. The result of this experience was similar to his attempt to synthesize the scurvy literature. He became confused and overwhelmed as he reviewed his own work. He became convinced that scurvy was due to putrefaction and then the blocking of perspiration. He recommended that lemon juice be mixed with wine and sugar. This led to an effervescent drink, which was helpful for the digestive system. He did continue to use lemons, sometimes with success. He described this in a balanced, careful, and unhelpful way: "I do not mean to say that lemon juice and wine are the only remedy for the scurvy; this disease, like many others, may be cured by medicines of very different, and opposite qualities to each other, and to that of lemons."[3] This is an astonishing sentence written by the man universally credited for discovering the citrus cure for scurvy.

Why did Lind never reproduce his *HMS Salisbury* results? There is no clear answer. Some have suggested that the sick sailors at Haslar knew that citrus fruits would help them, so all of Lind's Haslar experiments were ruined by the sailors managing to get hold of citrus fruit. This would mean that comparisons between different treatment groups would be misleading. Perhaps some sailors were ill with other diseases. Another possibility is that the lemon juice was adulterated or spoiled. On the *HMS Salisbury*, Lind used actual fruit. As we will see below, the change from fruit to fruit juice sometimes was accompanied by loss of the active vitamin.

Lind made many other suggestions about the welfare of sailors that were sensible and humane. He emphasized the importance of providing ventilated, warm, and dry quarters. He described ways of distilling seawater to produce drinkable water. He advocated regular exercise for the sailors. Finally, he made an astute observation about officers, sailors, and scurvy. The officers often thought that the fatigue that accompanied scurvy was just the laziness of the sailors. Sailors with scurvy who were forced to continue with hard physical labor often died. Thus, we see one of mankind's most unfortunate and common tendencies: to blame the sick for their illness or to attribute it to character defect. Lind was a man of many virtues, and his refusal to give in to this tendency was not the least of them. By the end of his life, Lind blamed the illness on cold damp air, confinement, and the "stoppage" of perspiration. The humors had defeated him.

Captain James Cook Measures the Transit of Venus, Looks for an Imaginary Continent, and Keeps His Sailors Healthy

Captain James Cook (1728–1779), the great explorer, was a contemporary of Lind. Like Lind, he had humble beginnings. He was born to a day laborer in Yorkshire, but he was very ambitious and saw at an early age that there were opportunities at sea. He began his career working for some years as an apprentice on a coal ship. He joined the Royal Navy as an "able seaman" and worked his way up the ranks. In 1763 he took command of the schooner *Grenville* and surveyed the eastern coasts of Canada and Newfoundland for four years. In 1768 an opportunity from the skies appeared. This was the transit of Venus, the passage of the planet between the Sun and the Earth. Venus was due to cross the Sun on June 3, 1769 and then not again for more than one hundred years. The Royal Geographic Society organized voyages so that the transit could be observed from various locations to help with calculations of the distance from the Earth to the Sun.

The Royal Society and Navy chose James Cook to command the voyage to the South Pacific. Cook was then still only a relatively minor sea captain but already respected for his seamanship, charting, mathematical, and geographical abilities displayed in his Canadian work. Cook was an inspired choice. In addition to his other skills, he also possessed great observational and psychological skills that would be very important in his later work. Cook left the chilly waters off Newfoundland for warmer coasts. Cook sailed the refitted coal bark, the *Endeavour*. He was assigned the task of taking astronomic measurements and also finding the supposed southern continent—*terra australis incognita*—in the South Pacific. The Ancient Greeks had thought that there must be a southern continent to "balance" the masses of the northern continents. This was a strange time for geographers. Scientists were attempting to describe the distance between the Earth and the Sun, while still being unsure of the continents of their own planet. Another research task assigned to Cook and the *Endeavour* was to investigate possible treatments for scurvy.

The *Endeavour* sailed to Tahiti, and Cook made multiple measurements of the transit of Venus. Once this was done he continued to search for the southern continent. He did not find this nonexistent continent, but he successfully charted numerous other islands, including the entire coastline of New Zealand. The voyage lasted from 1768 to 1771. Not a single sailor was lost to scurvy. He was the first naval commander not to have a long voyage marred by scurvy. In his second voyage he commanded the *Resolution* and was accompanied by another ship, the *Adventure*. Sailors on the *Resolution* stayed healthy, and sailors on the *Adventure* became ill. How did Cook keep his sailors scurvy free during these long trips? What was the difference between the *Resolution* and the *Adventure*? The difference lay in Cook's conviction that fresh food and preserved cabbage were important. Cook also appreciated the importance of leading by example. He understood that the sailors would not want to eat the sauerkraut:

> (I) had some of it dressed every day for the (officers') cabin table and left it to the option of the men either to take as much as they pleased or none at all; but . . . before a week I found it necessary to put every one on board to an allowance, for . . . whatever you give seamen out of the common way, although it be ever so much for their good yet . . . you will hear nothing but murmurings against the man that first invented it; but the moment they see their superiors set a value upon it, it becomes the finest stuff in the world and the inventor an honest fellow. . . .[4]

Cook took much experimental food on board with him, including sauerkraut and wort, a liquid made from barley, which was thought to be helpful for treating scurvy. He also insisted that the ship get fresh food at every port that he stopped at. One of his sailors noted that they were always praised by Cook if they were seen coming back to the ship with fresh vegetables.[5] Cook had done the right thing by his sailors, but his multiple approaches to good nutrition made it impossible to pin down the exact factor that prevented scurvy. It was difficult to determine whether it was fresh food, sauerkraut, or wort that had prevented the scurvy.

Gilbert Blane and the "Limey"

So far, we have shown that many sailors knew that citrus fruits or fresh vegetables prevented or treated scurvy but that this knowledge was lost. Lind rediscovered this in a simple and convincing trial, but no one read his description. Lind then lost his nerve and returned to blaming scurvy on a disarray of the humors. Cook was successful in preventing scurvy, but no one was quite sure how. The use of limes in the English navy is thanks to the work of a much less famous man. Gilbert Blane (1749–1834), another Scottish physician, was quite different from his countryman James Lind. He had less nautical experience but more prestige (at the time). He served only ten months with the Channel Fleet in 1780 as a physician and then left to set up a successful private practice in London. He was the personal physician of Lord George Rodney, an influential British admiral. Blane was not an original thinker or an experimenter, but he read Lind's book, and he understood the importance of Lind's trial. He read the medical documents and surgeons' reports from Cook's voyages. Blane synthesized what he read. Lind and Cook had become lost in their own experiences. Blane, having the advantage of some distance, did not. Blane also had the advantage of loving numbers.

Blane became convinced through his analyzing, collation, and formation of tables that the English navy must address the health of the sailors. More sailors were dying from infectious illnesses and scurvy than from enemy action. Blane noted, with bitterness, that the navy was more anxious about the condition of the ropes and gunpowder than the health of the sailors.[6] He concluded that the navy should provide citrus fruit to its sailors. In 1794, because of Blane's influence, all sailors on board the *Suffolk*, sailing to India, were issued two thirds of an ounce of lemon juice mixed in grog. No one developed scurvy. This was a more successful trip than the first trip from Europe to India, led by Vasco da Gama. Thanks to his friends in high places, Blane was appointed to be a Commissioner of the Board of the Sick and Wounded Sailors in 1795 and ordered that lemon juice be issued to all English sailors. More than forty years after Lind's trial, his findings were put into practice. Lime juice was often used instead of lemon juice, and the English sailor became known as the "limey." Over time, the term "limey" was often applied to any English person. Ironically, as we shall see later, lime juice has less anti-scurvy activity than lemon juice. Lind, despite his brilliance, was not an aggressive or persuasive man. Blane loved numbers, tables, and the company of lords. He was eloquent. Together, these dissimilar Scottish physicians led to one of the greatest advances in the English navy and medicine.[7]

The importance of lemon juice to the English navy can hardly be overstated. At the end of the eighteenth century, Napoleon Bonaparte (1769–1821) was planning to conquer Europe. He had large and well-trained armies and undoubtedly would have been able to defeat England had he been able to land in that country. The English navy organized a blockade of the English Channel to prevent the French fleet from crossing over to England. This blockade meant that British ships patrolled the English Channel continuously, often not putting into port for months at a time. The blockade lasted from 1795 to 1815. Without lemon or lime juice, the navy would not have had the manpower to be able to perform their duty.

Lord Horatio Nelson (1758–1805), a commander of the English navy, had suffered from scurvy himself as a young man; therefore, he took the illness very seriously. Not only did he comply with the new rules of the navy in supplying lemon juice to all sailors, but he went further. In February 1805 he had been issued thirty thousand gallons of lemon juice. He ordered a supplement of twenty thousand gallons for his Mediterranean fleet. At the Battle of Trafalgar on October 21, 1805, Lord Nelson and his scurvy-free sailors defeated Napoleon's navy. The Royal Navy was now the strongest fleet in the world, and Britain dominated global trade throughout the nineteenth century. Even though no one understood how citrus fruits were helpful, this should have been the end of scurvy in the English navy and indeed throughout the world, but problems remained. Scurvy afflicted British soldiers in Turkey, British explorers in the Arctic, and children of the wealthy in Britain and the United States.

Scurvy and the Crimean War: Cabbages Thrown into the Harbor

The Crimean War (1853–1856) was fought on the Crimean Peninsula in western Turkey. The war was the result of chronic tension between Europe and Russia. Russia had been expanding its empire south into the Ottoman Empire and was attempting to gain control of Constantinople and, with it, access to the Mediterranean. France, Turkey, and Britain were alarmed at the possible change in the balance of power. Disputes between the French and Russians about the control of Christian shrines in Jerusalem were the immediate cause of the war. This war was renowned for military follies, epitomized by the charge of the light brigade, which was memorialized by Alfred Lord Tennyson, but even more irresponsible than the military were the negligent supporting departments.

During the Crimean War, Florence Nightingale (1820–1910) rose to fame, in part for her confrontation of the bureaucratic quagmires. Britain sent her to Turkey in 1854 to tackle the deplorable care of the wounded. She faced many challenges: poor sanitation, inadequate food, and no way of delivering medical supplies. More soldiers died from infectious illnesses than battle wounds. The rigidity of military thinking often interfered with the care for the English soldier. For example, in 1854, news that the troops were suffering from scurvy reached England. Of twelve hundred sick soldiers at Scutari, most were ill with scurvy. The army arranged for lime juice and cabbages to be sent to the army. Woodham-Smith, biographer of Nightingale, describes what happened next:

> In January, 1855, when the army before Sebastopol was being ravaged by scurvy, a shipload of cabbages was thrown into the harbour at Balaclava on the ground that it was not consigned to anyone. This happened not once but several times . . . 20,000 lb. of lime-juice arrived for the troops on December 10, 1854, but none was issued until February. Why? Because no order existed for the inclusion of . . . lime-juice in the daily ration. . . .[8]

In other words, the acceptance of the food from the ships at Balaclava and the inclusion of lime juice in the diet were not clearly the responsibility of anyone, so they did not get done. Is it possible that the army did not understand the importance of getting these food items to the troops? Or were the various officers so entrenched in their various administrative roles that they were unable to take the necessary steps to ensure that the troops would not suffer from scurvy? The incompetence of the British commissary department had defeated the work of Lind and aided the Russian troops. Blane had emphasized how important it was to care for the British *sailor*, but this did not apparently apply to the British *soldier*. This is similar to the situation in Japan described earlier. Takaki's discovery of the importance of nutrition for the Japanese navy was ignored by the Japanese army.

Advances in science and medicine can be thwarted by bureaucratic inertia. Individuals in the British commissary department would not have murdered individual British soldiers, but their sloth in ensuring that cabbages and lime juice be delivered to the British troops in Scutari killed the troops as surely as did Russian bullets. Nightingale, in a characteristically sarcastic vein, wrote that the Crimean War and treatment of the British soldier were an experiment in seeing how many men could die because of filth and poor food.[9]

Arctic Exploration and Scurvy: Finding the Northwest Passage

The mysterious polar regions of the Earth tempted explorers who were exposed to tribulations that we can barely imagine today. One of the worst was scurvy. Why would people voluntarily travel to these frozen lands? The reason was that travel in the Arctic was a way of gaining great fame and riches. Merchants and explorers were convinced that there was a strait or waterway through North America that would allow a quick and easy passage from Europe to the Pacific Ocean and the treasures beyond. Some believed in the existence of a warm polar sea, which would be a particularly easy Northwest Passage. The idea of a Northwest Passage was alluring to Europeans for the next four centuries.

The actual search for a Northwest Passage proved to be anything but quick and easy. Travelers in search of the Northwest Passage had to cope with subzero temperatures, drifting and shifting icepacks, howling storms, unpredictable calving icebergs, and impassable glaciers. A strait that had been easy to sail through just twelve months before would be frozen over on a return journey. The Arctic ice pack was equally capricious. The explorers could be trapped on ice floes which could drift in any direction, often in the direction opposite to the one the explorers would have wished. The explorers faced isolation, injuries, boredom, and long Arctic nights. When the sun did appear, during the pitifully short Arctic summers, it led to snow blindness. Their travails have been described, often in gruesome detail. The more gruesome the detail, the better selling the accounts would be.

A major problem was always the supply of food, particularly because the extreme cold increased the need for calories. Travelers carried food with them, but the supply could be exhausted because of bad planning, unforeseen accidents, or delays. If the travelers ran out of food, they could hunt deer, reindeer, seals, or polar bears if they were willing or capable. In later trips, when dogs joined the expeditions, the travelers would eat their own dogs. In some cases, there may have been cannibalism. Yet, the Arctic was not unpopulated. Groups of Inuit, or Eskimos, lived there. Eskimos never suffered from scurvy, even though they rarely ate fresh fruit or vegetables. Pierre Berton, the great Canadian documenter of the North, describes this surprising situation in his retelling of the expeditions of Sir William Parry (1790–1855), one of the celebrated Arctic explorers. Parry led a number of unsuccessful expeditions to the Arctic in search of the elusive Northwest Passage between 1818 and 1828 and saw many cases of scurvy among his men:

> Most puzzling of all, and most damning, is that in an age of science Europeans were unable to understand how the Eskimos escaped the great Arctic scourge that struck almost every white expedition to the North. The seeds of scurvy were already in Parry's men, in spite of the lemon juice and marmalade, but no one connected the Eskimos' diet with the state of their health . . . the explorers sensed that scurvy was linked to diet and that fresh meat and vegetables helped ward it off . . . Nobody caught on to the truth that raw meat and blubber are effective antiscorbutics [anti-scurvy agents]. For another half century, the Navy sent ship after ship into the North loaded down with barrels of salt meat while Navy cooks boiled or roasted away all the vitamins from the fresh provisions that were sometimes available.
>
> Why this apparent blindness? Part of it, no doubt, was the conservatism of the senior service and part of the arrogance of the nineteenth century English upper classes, who considered themselves superior to most other peoples. . . .[10]

The British felt that they must act properly at all times and never take up the customs of the indigenous people. They wore clothes and shoes that were comically unfitted for Arctic travel. They used tents and traveled with heavy sleds that they pulled themselves, thinking that the Eskimo use of dogs was cruel.

They could not understand why the Eskimos or Indians dressed the way they did or ate what they did. The idea that the native peoples would have known what they were doing did not occur to the English.

In contrast to the English were the French-Canadian voyageurs who worked for companies such as the Hudson Bay Company and other fur trading concerns. They manned canoes carrying goods and supplies that were traded in exchange for furs. They often served as guides for explorers. The voyageurs had no difficulty copying the customs of the natives. They understood the sense of dressing in furs, eating off the land, and traveling lightly. The English looked down on these men. One exception to this story of English arrogance and folly is Sir James Clark Ross (1800–1862). He spent four winters trapped in the Arctic. Yet, like Cook, he was remarkable in that he brought his crew back home with few losses to scurvy. He attributed his success to paying careful attention to the diet of the Eskimos.

As we saw with Jacques Cartier, the indigenous people of North America had much to teach the explorers. Cartier and his men were able to consume drinks made from bark and leaves, and Sir Ross was able to learn to eat what the Eskimos did. But most of the Arctic explorers found bear, musk oxen, or seal, sometimes frozen or rotten, too different or too odiferous to eat.

Scurvy and the Franklin and Nares Expeditions

Problems with food supply plagued even the most famous and lavishly prepared exhibition—that of Sir John Franklin. Franklin (1786–1847) had served in the Royal Navy since the age of fourteen. He had taken part in many famous battles, including the Battle of Trafalgar in 1805 and the Battle of New Orleans in 1814. The Royal Navy (and Franklin) faced a new danger after Napoleon was defeated at Waterloo in 1815. The navy was in danger of becoming obsolete. The officers were underemployed and were losing opportunities for promotion. The navy turned its energies to polar exploration. Franklin went north. He was second in command of a sea voyage into the Arctic. He commanded an overland expedition that surveyed much of the shoreline of the Canadian tundra in 1819. During this expedition, ten men died from cold and hunger. He returned to the north for another overland expedition in 1825.

Then, he served the Royal Navy in the Mediterranean, and after that, he was appointed governor of Van Diemen's Land, a penal colony off the south coast of Australia. He governed there for six years and did so exceptionally badly. Part of the problem was his wife, Lady Jane Franklin, who was despised in Van Diemen's Land for her autocratic and aristocratic ways. He was finally recalled to England, where yet another expedition to seek the Northwest Passage was being formed. Lady Jane Franklin, his indomitable wife, begged that her husband be considered for this expedition. She must have hoped that he could gain glory in the northern end of the Earth to make up for his disgrace at the southern end. Due in part to Lady Franklin's pleading and despite the concerns of some about Sir Franklin's age (fifty-eight) and physical condition (plump), he was put in charge of the expedition. The expedition boasted technologically advanced ships (the *Erebus* and the *Terror*). They had sails, but they also had steam-powered engines and iron plating. Both ships had already traveled to the Antarctic. They were further strengthened with iron plating and additional African oak and Canadian fir and elm.

The ships were stocked with plentiful provisions. This trip took place after the work of Lind had been recognized by Blane, so the navy knew about the importance of vegetables and fruit. The new invention of canning food was expected to solve the problem of scurvy. The Admiralty ordered over nine thousand gallons of lemon juice and five tons of pickles, cabbages, onions, and cranberries. Over two tons of dried peas and dried apples, dates, and canned milk were loaded onto the ships. The food, much of it precooked, was preserved in airtight tins, which also protected the food from rats. The food was enough to last the expedition for three years.

The Franklin expedition left England in May 1845 with 129 men to search for the Northwest Passage in the labyrinth of the Arctic Archipelago. They met two whaling ships in Baffin Bay in July 1845. Nobody ever saw Franklin or his crew again. No other large expeditionary force had disappeared so completely as had Franklin and his sailors. Lady Jane Franklin became an international heroine by refusing to believe that her husband and his crew had perished. Perhaps she felt guilty that she was in large part responsible for her husband's voyage. She pleaded with the British government again—this time, to send out more expeditions to search for him. She wrote letters to the new emperor of France and to the tsar of Russia. She engendered much sympathy and support. More than fifty expeditions scoured the Arctic over the next fourteen years looking for Sir Franklin and his 128 men. Berton wrote that ". . . the main cause of death was clearly scurvy. Franklin himself would succumb earlier than most of the others, perhaps as a result of the infirmities of age. But the remaining crew, almost to a man, dropped in their tracks, their gums blackened, their teeth rattling loosely in their heads, their flesh spongy and sunken from internal bleeding—weakened, debilitated. . . ."[11]

The generous food supply caused problems for Franklin because of its provenance. The Admiralty had put out bids for over forty-five tons of food. The provisions came from the stores of a Stephen Goldner, who had made the lowest bid. Goldner delivered several hundred thousand cans just days before the ships left. The timing made it impossible for the navy to examine the cans. The cans were flawed in many ways. They were insufficiently heated to kill *Clostridium* spores, the cause of botulism. They were badly soldered so that many burst, and the solder was toxic arsenic and lead. What was in the cans was of no higher quality than the cans themselves. The soup was diluted, the vegetables were unwashed, and the meat often was only gristle, skin, offal, bones, and excrement.

The problems with Goldner's supplies were, at least in part, because of his outright knavery and skill in cheating the Admiralty. Some of the ease in cheating the Admiralty was due to the novelty of canned food and the inexperience of the Admiralty in knowing how to deal with this new kind of food. There was little quality assurance or supervision of his buying or canning. Years later, after much more painful experience with Goldner and evidence against him from his own employees, the navy stopped buying food from him. Franklin's expedition relied on the canned food. The food represented a choice between Scylla and Charybdis. Some of the canned food—such as Goldner's pickles, vegetables, raisins, and gooseberries—might have staved off scurvy. However, the canned food might have caused deaths through lead poisoning and botulism. Once the canned food ran out, the men stopped dying from the diseases caused by the canned food, but they developed scurvy. Sir John Franklin and his men might have fared better had they been provided with less food and more encouragement to live "off the land," but the expedition was not supplied with any means of hunting deer, polar bear, or seals, which would have provided them with Vitamin C.

One more expedition to the Arctic was to suffer from scurvy, although with less disastrous circumstances. George Nares (1831–1915) was put in charge of another expedition to discover the North Pole. This expedition set off in 1875 and was provided with lime juice. Scurvy once again developed and ruined the expedition. It was not clear why Nares' men developed scurvy, but he was reprimanded harshly. Later investigations would lead to the probable reason for scurvy in this expedition and exonerate Nares.

Infantile Scurvy

There was one unexpected group of people whose health was generally good—except for scurvy—the children of the wealthy or educated. In the late 1800s, cases of scurvy in children in the United States and England began to be reported. Autopsies of these children showed dramatic changes in their bones. The tissue around the bone was separated from the bone itself by blood clots, and this may have caused the pain often suffered by these children. Why were these children developing scurvy?

Scurvy in children was an unintended consequence of one of the greatest health advances of the time. Until the late nineteenth century, milk from cows was often adulterated and/or contaminated with blood, mucus, pus, and dung. Drinking milk led to a number of illnesses, including typhoid fever, scarlet fever, diphtheria, diarrheal diseases, and bovine tuberculosis.

FEEDING COW MILK TO INFANTS

Human breast milk is the natural food for infants, but cow milk is a common alternative. The value of the cow milk depends on how well fed and healthy the cows are, how cleanly the milk is collected, and how quickly the cow milk is transported to the infant. Raw milk easily spoils and in the past often caused illnesses.

Pasteurization of milk was introduced in the late 1800s as a way of decreasing milk-borne illnesses and was successful, but the pasteurization led to unforeseen problems. In 1914, a pediatrician in New York, Alfred Hess, noticed scurvy in some of his young patients who were otherwise well. They were drinking pasteurized milk. He was able to treat them by adding raw milk, orange juice, or potatoes to their diet. (Hess is discussed further in the Vitamin D chapter.) It seemed that pasteurization, although clearly helpful in combating bacterial contamination, did have the side effect of being associated with scurvy.

Axel Holst, Theodor Frölich, and the Guinea Pig

Lind's experiment showed that oranges and lemons were good *treatment* for the disease. His experiment was elegant, simple, and conclusive, but it did not prove that citrus fruit deficiency *caused* the illness. The proof that scurvy was a deficiency disease—that Bachstrom and Cocchi had been right all along—came from a Norwegian laboratory using experimental animals. The work was done on the guinea pig.

Axel Holst (1860–1931), a Norwegian professor of hygiene and bacteriology, like so many eminent researchers of the time, had worked in Koch's laboratory in Germany. He had also worked at the Pasteur Institute and had visited Eijkman's laboratory in the Dutch East Indies. He was interested in both infectious and dietary causes of illness. He and his colleagues were investigating outbreaks of "ship beriberi" in the Norwegian shipping fleet. He and Theodore Frölich, a Norwegian biochemist, followed Eijkman's example and worked with pigeons. They were unable to produce the illness that resembled the Norwegian problem of ship beriberi. They then switched animals and began to work with guinea pigs. They found that guinea pigs became ill when fed diets of just a single grain.

Examination of the dead guinea pigs showed hemorrhages, looseness of the teeth, and bone fragility. The changes in the bones and cartilage were similar to those in autopsies performed on children with scurvy. The guinea pig had developed scurvy. This was a new finding. Until this time, scurvy had not been clearly described in animals. This was not the illness that the Norwegians were studying, but they had the nimbleness and intelligence to seize on this unexpected opportunity. They began to study scurvy.

How is it that guinea pigs were used by the Norwegian scientists?

These two Norwegian physicians had chosen one of the few animals that needs Vitamin C. The rodent from the Andes has a strange human-like inability to synthesize this vitamin. Rats and pigeons, other commonly used laboratory animals, synthesize their own Vitamin C, so work with them could never have led to the discovery.

Holst and Frölich experimented with feeding their guinea pigs different foods. The guinea pigs stayed healthy if fed fresh potatoes but became ill and died when fed dried potatoes. Cabbage prevented scurvy. This explained, in

---

GUINEA PIGS

The guinea pig is neither a pig, nor from Guinea. It is a rodent, whose scientific name is *Cavia porcellus*. The word "cavia" comes from Quechua, the language of the Incas. The Andean people raised guinea pigs as livestock and named them cui, or cuy, possibly after the squeals of the animals. The rodent is small, plump, and slow moving. It is fertile and raises multiple litters. The cuy is a friendly and docile rodent that does not bite humans. The cuy was kept in homes of the Andeans and raised both for consumption and as a pet.

Oviedo, a chronicler who accompanied the conquistador Francisco Pizarro to the Andes, named the rodent *"chancito de la India"* (*chancito* is Spanish for pig), possibly because of its squeals or possibly because it reminded him of European pigs that were sometimes kept in houses, fed on scraps, and then eaten themselves. The *chancito* was brought back to Europe. It became known as "guinea pig"—the derivation of the "guinea" is not known. Queen Elizabeth I (1533–1603) is reported to have had one as a pet.

Because of its small size and good nature, the guinea pig was a good experimental animal. Antoine Lavoisier (1743–1794), the great French chemist, used them in his work with respiration. Robert Koch used them in his studies of microbes and infection. Guinea pigs proved to be susceptible to developing tuberculosis. These qualities were fortunate for the experimenter and less so for the rodent.

---

part, Cook's success on his trips to the South Pacific when he encouraged his men to eat sauerkraut. The Norwegians could *cause* scurvy and *treat* it by manipulating the diet of the guinea pigs. Holst and Frölich published their results in 1907. Scurvy was not an infectious disease or a toxic process. Scurvy was a dietary deficiency disease.

Lemons and Sweet and Sour Limes

The work of Holst and Frölich provided other scientists with an animal model for scurvy. The Norwegian work was used to great effect by Harriette Chick (1875–1977), one of the century's great nutritionists. She had trained as a bacteriologist and had studied in Munich and Vienna. She returned from Europe to work at the Lister Institute in London with plague and fleas. Her career was changed by World War I. Many male physicians were fighting in the war, so her gender, rather than holding her back as it might have otherwise done, in fact protected her. Also, the war meant that experts in nutrition were needed. Soldiers needed to be fed, as did civilian populations living in war-ravaged communities. (We shall meet Chick again in the Vitamin D chapter.)

In 1915, Chick was taken away from the plague and put in charge of the task of identifying food that could support the English troops overseas. Once again, the English army was in trouble in Turkey. The Battle of Gallipoli took place in Turkey between April and December of 1915. This was quite different from the Crimean War, in that this time, the British and Ottoman Empires were enemies. British, French, Indian, and Australian troops attempted to capture Istanbul and failed. During this battle, troops faced terrible conditions, and many troops became ill with diseases such as amoebic dysentery and malaria. They were also badly fed, and many troops became ill with beriberi and scurvy. To provide as much practical advice as possible for the troops and aware of the work of Holst and Frölich, Chick and her team worked with guinea pigs. They fed the rodents a basic diet of oats, bran, and water and added items one at a time to see which ones prevented scurvy from developing. They were scrupulous in their techniques; as a result, they made a series of important discoveries.

Chick's team discovered that citrus fruits vary in how much anti-scurvy activity they had. Lemons had more anti-scurvy activity than limes, and Mediterranean sweet limes had more than West Indian sour limes. Limes could be bought from British Caribbean colonies. Lemons came from a non-British area, the Mediterranean. The Admiralty, not surprisingly, preferred limes. This discovery was illuminating. It explained some of the failures of lime juice to prevent scurvy and the disasters that had struck the Nares Arctic expeditions. Switching the type of citrus fruit from lemon to lime or sweet to sour lime was an important decision with bad consequences. Nares was not to blame for scurvy; the blame lay with the decision to switch from Mediterranean lemons to West Indian limes.[12]

Does Milk Prevent Scurvy?

Chick also discovered that fresh milk prevented the guinea pigs from developing scurvy, but this work was not replicated by one of her American nutritional colleagues. McCollum was doing his own experiments in Wisconsin with guinea pigs with scurvy and found that in his laboratory, fresh milk did not prevent scurvy. McCollum's rats did well on a diet of oats and milk alone, and he found it difficult to understand how a guinea pig, another rodent, could be so different. Searching for an explanation, he focused on the sluggish bowels of the guinea pig. McCollum came up with a rather old-fashioned theory as to the cause of scurvy—constipation.

What was the difference? Was English milk different from American milk? The difference turned out to lie elsewhere. Guinea pigs were like Cook's English sailors or Eijkman's Dutch chickens—they had to be cajoled to consume what was good for them. Chick and her team took a personal interest in making sure that the milk was consumed by the guinea pigs. They hand-fed the rodents, and they measured the amounts of milk consumed by the rodents. In Wisconsin, the guinea pigs were cared for by people who, not appreciating the importance of the milk, supplied the guinea pigs with milk and then went home for the weekend.

McCollum had discovered Vitamin A and was a part of the team that discovered Vitamin D, but he missed Vitamin C. He understood the importance of palatable diets for rodents but underestimated the importance of hand-feeding and was misled by his constipated guinea pigs. Other surprises followed. Scientists working in Holst's laboratories had made the important finding that some seeds had no anti-scurvy activity until they germinate. These findings were confirmed by Harriette Chick and her team. Peas and lentils were soaked for one day, and then germinated. In three days, these pulses acquired the ability to prevent scurvy.

Other researchers determined that any anti-scurvy activity was easily destroyed by heating. This important and unexpected finding explained the connection between scurvy and pasteurized milk. Chick's guinea pigs were fed unpasteurized milk, which had some anti-scurvy activity. Her rodents would not have responded so well to heated, or pasteurized, milk. This heat sensitivity also explained the disappointing results often encountered with some kinds of fruit juices. Fresh fruit was expensive, bulky, heavy, and not always available. On long sea journeys in those prerefrigeration days, fresh fruit or fresh juice was impractical. Some authorities thought, not unreasonably, that preserved fruit juice could be helpful. The best way of preserving fruit juice was to boil it into a syrup, but this meant that the anti-scurvy activity was lost. "Rob," a heated and condensed form of citrus juice, recommended with some trepidation by James Lind, probably contained very little anti-scurvy activity.

Some populations never eat fresh fruits, yet are without scurvy. The best example of this is the Eskimo population. This is due to their consumption of raw or minimally cooked meat. Vilhjalmur Stefansson (1879–1962) was a Canadian anthropologist and explorer who spent much time in the far north of Canada. He believed that the dangers and perils of travel in the north were much exaggerated. He wrote a book, *The Friendly Arctic*, to emphasize this. He ate a diet of lightly cooked meat for nine months and did well. By not cooking the meat too much, the anti-scurvy activity was not broken down.

The Naming of Vitamin C

In 1920, Sir Jack Drummond was Professor of Biochemistry at University College London and working with vitamins. As a young man, he had worked with Funk at the Lister Institute. Drummond saw that the anti-scurvy factor fit the description of what Funk described as "vitamines" in every way—except one. The factor was not an "amine." The anti-scurvy factor was an acidic carbohydrate. Drummond was the person who cleverly changed the name to vitamin by removing the final "e." McCollum had already used A and B to describe what he referred to as "factors." Drummond suggested that retinol and thiamine retain the letters of the alphabet to identify them, as Vitamins A and B, and that the anti-scurvy factor be named Vitamin C, and so it was.

Structure and Synthesis of Vitamin C, Formerly Known as "Ignose" or "Godnose" or "Hexuronic Acid"

Albert Szent-Györgyi (1893–1986), a member of an aristocratic Hungarian family, was brought up in Budapest, where he began medical school. He switched to research and then enrolled in the Hungarian army as a medic. He fought bravely in World War I but then became appalled by the carnage and extricated himself from the battlefields by shooting himself in the arm. In 1927 he went to England to study biochemistry with Hopkins. He found a new crystal in oranges, lemons, cabbages, and adrenal glands. Showing his irreverent nature, he named this new crystal "ignose." The "ose" referred to the chemical term for sugar. The entire word indicated that he did not know what it was exactly. He submitted an article about "ignose" to the *Biochemical Journal.* The editor was not amused. Szent-Györgyi tried again. He named his new substance "godnose." The editor remained unamused. Szent-Györgyi finally named the new molecule "hexuronic acid" because it had six carbons, and his article was published. Szent-Györgyi returned to Hungary in 1931. In a happy accident, he found himself in a laboratory surrounded by fields of red peppers in which there was abundant Vitamin C. Hexuronic acid and Vitamin C turned out to be the same molecule. Szent-Györgyi described its structure and received the 1937 Nobel Prize in Physiology or Medicine for this work.

STRUCTURE OF VITAMIN C

Vitamin C is made up of only three elements: six carbons, eight hydrogens, and six oxygens. Its chemical structure is similar to that of glucose, a simple sugar. Deficiency of this small molecule leads to the complicated illness scurvy. Its name, ascorbic acid, is a simpler form of the word first proposed by Dr. Johannes Bachstrom in 1734.

As so often happens with Nobel Prizes, this was controversial because another team, headed by the American Charles Glen King, had also performed this task. Vedder, who was involved in the discovery of thiamine, also discovered the structure of the vitamin independently. Szent-Györgyi was active in the Hungarian antifascist underground in World War II and played an important role in Hungarian politics after the war. He became disenchanted with the Soviet regime and moved to the United States in 1947, where he continued to do respected laboratory work for some years. In his later years, he became interested in more esoteric topics, such as the relationship between quantum physics and cancer. These interests, in contrast to his work on Vitamin C, were looked on skeptically by the scientific community.

Sir Walter Norman Haworth in Birmingham and the Polish chemist Tadeus Reichstein synthesized Vitamin C in 1934 simultaneously and independently. Haworth won the 1937 Nobel Prize in Chemistry for his work with Vitamin C. He shared this prize with Paul Karrer, who had worked with a number of other vitamins, including Vitamin A. Vitamin C was the first vitamin to be synthesized in the laboratory. Synthetic Vitamin C was proven to work by giving it to guinea pigs. Reichstein took out patents with Hoffman-LaRoche. Three Nobel Prizes were awarded to vitamin researchers in 1937, a banner year for nutrition:

- Albert Szent-Györgyi. Physiology or Medicine, for the discovery of the structure of Vitamin C.
- Walter Norman Haworth. Chemistry, for the synthesis of Vitamin C.
- Paul Karrer. Chemistry, for work on the structure of several vitamins.

(Reichstein was not ignored by Stockholm. He won a Nobel Prize in 1950 for his work with adrenal cortex hormones such as cortisone.)

Linus Pauling and Vitamin C

Linus Pauling (1901–1994) was an extraordinary man who was active in the areas of physics, chemistry, hematology, psychiatry, and politics. He won two Nobel Prizes, as an individual, in unrelated fields—a singular feat. He won his first Nobel Prize in Chemistry in 1954 for his work in characterizing the nature of chemical bonds. He was intrigued by X-ray crystallography and the importance of understanding the structure of proteins. Pauling discovered the important alpha helix, the shape of many proteins.

STRUCTURE OF PROTEINS

Proteins are made up of a string, or chain, of amino acids. The string folds into three-dimensional shapes. The shape of the protein determines how it will interact with other molecules. Pauling discovered one of the common ways of folding: the alpha helix. In the alpha helix, the chain of amino acids is coiled like a spring. The "backbone" of the peptide forms the inner part of the coil, whereas the side chains extend outward from the coil. The helix is stabilized by "hydrogen bonds" that were first described by Pauling.

He worked as a chemist at the California Institute of Technology, also known as Caltech. Pursuing his interest in structure and after a conversation with William Castle, he studied the shape of hemoglobin in sickle cell anemia. (Hemoglobin is described further in the chapter about Vitamins B9 and B12.) In this illness, the actual structure of the protein, hemoglobin, is altered by the substitution of one amino acid in a structure containing almost six hundred amino acids. This one change makes the red blood cell, mostly composed of hemoglobin, become sickle-shaped rather than concave at low oxygen levels. The sickle-shaped cells "stick" in small vessels and cause much pain and damage. An understanding of the molecular structure of hemoglobin explained the clinical findings of this illness. Sickle cell anemia was one of the first diseases shown to be due to an abnormal human molecule.

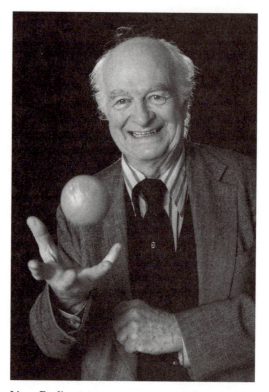

Linus Pauling tosses an orange, a good source of
Vitamin C, up into the air. © Roger Ressmeyer/
CORBIS.

Pauling was involved in politics, taking many controversial positions. The
U.S. State Department at times delayed granting him or renewing his passport
because of his left-wing activities. Without a passport, he was unable sometimes to attend international meetings. The FBI became interested in Pauling's
politics. The FBI monitored his political activities for twenty-five years and
compiled a twenty-five-hundred-page file about him. His campaigning against
nuclear testing annoyed the conservative trustees of Caltech. Caltech believed
that he should be more active in chemistry and less active in protest. Despite
his lack of popularity with the State Department, FBI, and Caltech, he was
awarded the 1962 Nobel Peace Prize for his work in organizing international
campaigns to ban nuclear bomb testing. The Nobel Peace Prize did not pacify
the trustees of Caltech; shortly after he was awarded it, Pauling left Caltech.

Pauling became interested in Vitamin C in 1966 after meeting Irwin Stone
(1907–1984), an American biochemist. Stone had become interested in the
vitamin after working with it as a food preservative. He believed that humans
needed to consume it in large amounts. Pauling suffered with severe colds
and sinus infections and often was treated with penicillin. Following Stone's

advice, he took high doses of Vitamin C and believed that as a consequence, he got fewer colds and was able to stop taking penicillin. Other researchers carried out a number of studies to test this theory. The consensus was that Vitamin C is modestly effective in lowering the number of days that one is ill with a cold. Few researchers found that Vitamin C was as effective as Pauling and Stone believed it to be.

He became interested in Vitamin C and cancer in 1971 after learning of the results of a Scottish surgeon. Ewan Cameron (1922–1991) treated some of his patients with terminal cancer with large doses of Vitamin C and reported that high doses of Vitamin C prolonged their life. Other physicians tested high doses of Vitamin C in their patients with cancer and did not get the same results. Pauling and Cameron argued that the trials were not performed correctly. Pauling also became interested in the possibility of vitamins, particularly niacin, being used in the treatment of psychiatric disorders. This is discussed in the Vitamin B3 chapter.

Summary of Pauling's Contributions to Medicine

Pauling's explanation of the molecular cause of sickle cell anemia was a major contribution to medicine. His brilliant conceptions of the hydrogen bond, alpha helix, and X-ray crystallography advanced our understanding of molecular biology. His work with the treatments of cancer, psychiatric illness, and the common cold has not been clinically useful so far. His investigations into Vitamin C and niacin have brought much public attention to these vitamins, but also much medical skepticism. As he demonstrated in his persistent and highly unpopular work discouraging nuclear test bans, Pauling never minded pursuing a line of action that was not accepted by the "establishment."

SUMMARY

The history of scurvy reveals man at his most adventurous, traveling across stormy seas far from the comforts and fruits of dry land, and at his most fractious, fighting strangers for the possession of religious shrines or foreign cities. To support these activities, a simple sugar-like molecule is needed. Much observation suggested that citrus fruits provided this molecule. Laboratory work with the chubby and unfortunate guinea pig and the Hungarian pepper confirmed this answer. Work in the London Lister Institute laboratories revealed important information about this elegant molecule: Vitamin C is not sturdy.

6

Soft Bones, Lack of Light, and the "Sunshine Hormone": Vitamin D (Calcitriol), the Anti-Rickets Vitamin

Overview

Working out the cause of rickets was the path to the discovery of Vitamin D. In the past, children in cities or northern latitudes had soft bones. This was rickets, also known as "the English Disease," and it became more common during the industrial revolution that began in England in the late 1700s. Rickets is easily recognizable because of its distinct features. The child with rickets is typically a toddler with bowed legs or knock knees, splayed-out wrists, and knobs along their breastbone, known as the rachitic rosary. The rickety child also may develop slowly and experience bone pains.

In the early twentieth century, two researchers discovered independently that ultraviolet radiation from the sun can cure rickets. At the same time, it was known that cod-liver oil prevented and cured the illness. A trio of scientists showed that irradiation of sterols, molecules in cell membranes, led to the anti-rickets vitamin. Later, scientists showed that the vitamin protects us from a host of chronic illnesses. We do not need to eat foods with Vitamin D—as long as we are exposed to ultraviolet radiation that changes a cholesterol-like molecule in our skin to the vitamin. Without sunshine, which contains within it this invisible radiation, we must consume Vitamin D from foods such as cod-liver oil or from other foods fortified with synthetic Vitamin D. The importance of Vitamin D is greater than its contribution to the mineralization of bones. It is a hormone that acts throughout the body to regulate cell growth and forestall the development of some autoimmune illnesses and cancers.

Rickets in the Past

In 1650, Francis Glisson, an English physician, described rickets and wrote that it was most common in children between the age of six months and two and a half years. He was not sure of the cause, but he had ideas about treatment. He suggested cautery, incisions, and blistering. To correct

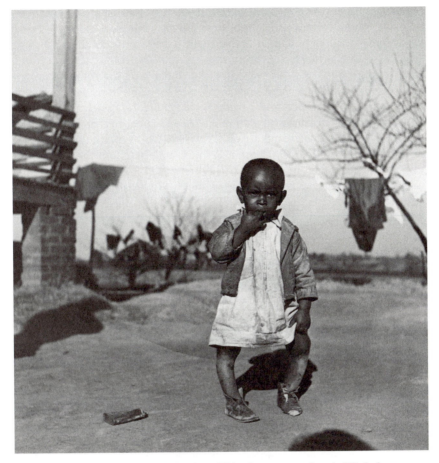

Child shows bowed legs typical of rickets. This picture was taken in Wadesboro, North Carolina, in December 1938. © Marion Post Wolcott/CORBIS.

the bony deformity, he suggested that the child be suspended in the air in an odd contraption that would stretch out the body and thus straighten the bones.[1]

As with many other illnesses, the exact cause of rickets was difficult to pin down. It was blamed on a variety of causes—dirty clothes, lack of exercise, poor sanitation, and syphilis. Despite this, some remarkable physicians had a sense of the cause and cure. In the middle of the nineteenth century, Armand Trousseau (1801–1867), a French physician, wrote that rickets in infancy and osteomalacia (soft bones) in adults were the same illness. He suggested that cold or sunless climates or poor diet caused the illness. He recommended the correct treatment—cod-liver (or any fish) oil, or prolonged breastfeeding, as long as the mother's milk was good, or exposure to sunlight.

Jedrzej Sniadecki (1768–1838), a Polish doctor, saw that children in Warsaw were more likely to suffer from rickets than were children in the Polish countryside. He thought that lack of sunshine was the cause of this difference. He took children with rickets from the city into the countryside and their rickets disappeared. Another physician who understood the role of sunshine in rickets was Theobald Palm, a medical representative from the Edinburgh Missionary Medical Society. As a medical missionary, he traveled throughout the world. Rickets in countries with abundant sunshine was rare, but in large cities in England and Scotland, it was common. Palm sent out questionnaires to his fellow missionaries in China and Tibet, and, based on the answers he received, he concluded in 1890 that children raised in filthy homes on poor food did not develop rickets—as long as they were breastfed and spent time in the sun.

The conclusions of Trousseau, Sniadecki, and Palm were correct, but their work had little impact, perhaps because it was ahead of its time or not published in widely read journals. The idea that sunlight or cod-liver oil could help form the bones of children was difficult to grasp. Just like the cure for scurvy that was known but lost, the cure for rickets became a relic of the past that was relegated to the wastebasket of folklore or old wives' tales.

The Sun Disappears, Rickets Becomes More Common

Rickets became common in the northern industrial cities in the eighteenth century because of the industrial revolution. The new mechanical inventions needed power, which, over time, came from the burning of coal. Coal was plentiful in England, cheap, reliable, and a highly concentrated source of energy. Industrial boilers burned coal to produce steam, which powered much of the machinery of the industrial revolution. Byproducts of burning coal, such as sulfur dioxide and other emissions, produced the infamous London smogs of the nineteenth and twentieth centuries. The particles in the air caused irritation to lungs and blocked both visible and invisible radiation from the sun. The London smog was an effective sun screen.

Labor moved from the home to the factory. Work became mechanized and centralized. Large factories were built, and children as young as six or seven were recruited to work there, for the same reasons that they were hired in the cotton mills in the southern United States. They worked long hours—often twelve to fourteen hours a day for six days a week. Children who worked in the English factories seldom saw the sun.

Many children in industrial cities throughout Europe and the United States—not just England—in the eighteenth to early twentieth centuries developed rickets. The situation was even worse for younger children. Toddlers are most at risk for becoming ill with rickets because bones form so rapidly during the ages of six to twenty-four months.

GREENSTICK FRACTURES

Without Vitamin D, a child's bones do not contain enough calcium; therefore, they break or fracture easily. These are known as greenstick fractures because of the similarity with bending a young branch. As the child begins to walk and put weight on a rickety bone, one side of the bone breaks, and the other deforms. Bones heal, but in a bended way. The child becomes bowlegged or knock-kneed.

The situation was worse for African American children in large cities in the United States because their pigmentation was another barrier to sunshine. At the beginning of the twentieth century, almost every African American toddler living in the North suffered with rickets.

Inadequate Diet: Lessons from the London Zoo

Cod-liver oil had been known to be a healthy food for many years in fishing communities along the coasts of northern Europe. For example, in the north of Scotland, cod-liver oil was often given to the ill and highly valued as a healthy food. Not many other people willingly eat this food, yet in Scotland, it was considered a delicacy. Supporting evidence for the nutritional benefits of cod-liver oil came from an unexpected venue—the tropical animal section at the London Zoo. This section had major problems in the late 1800s. The lions mated, conceived, and bore young, but the cubs did not survive. During one period at the London Zoo, more than twenty litters of cubs developed extreme rickets and died.

In 1889, Bland-Sutton, an English anatomist and surgeon with an interest in diseases of animals, became involved. He made some pertinent observations about the diet of the cubs. He noted that the cubs were fed lean meat. This seemed wrong to him because, in their natural habitat, lions do not just eat part of their prey. They eat small animals whole, including their organs and bones. Bland-Sutton suggested that the cub diet be changed to include bones, milk, and the remedy of northern European fishermen—cod-liver oil. This new diet was probably much closer to the diet that they received in the wild. The cubs thrived on this new diet. Bland-Sutton's observations about leonine rickets were seized on avidly by researchers of human rickets. (Bland-Sutton was a Victorian gentleman with an interest in the exotic and unconventional. He recreated a Persian chamber in his own house at one third the original size, popularized the hysterectomy, and invited people into the operating room to watch him operate.)

Puppies Eat "Scottish" Food and Frolic Outdoors

Hopkins, the originator of the concept of "accessory factors," recommended to the newly formed English Medical Research Committee that the task of solving rickets be assigned to a young scientist. As a result, in 1914,

Edward Mellanby (1884–1955), a student of Hopkins, began to work with puppies. He kept them indoors and fed them a diet consisting exclusively of porridge made from oats. This was known as the "Scottish diet." The dogs became rickety. Mellanby supplemented the diet of the puppies with yeast or orange juice, to no avail. He then showed that the dogs could be cured by the addition of butterfat or cod-liver oil to their diet. Mellanby was not sure what it was in the butterfat or cod-liver oil that hardened the canine bones. He thought that it might be McCollum's Vitamin A.

However, some critics thought that Mellanby had misunderstood his findings by not realizing the conditions in which the puppies had been kept. Other investigators found that puppies kept outside and allowed to exercise did not develop rickets, no matter what their diet. These critics suggested that Mellanby was wrong to blame rickets on nutritional problems and suggested, instead, that fresh air and exercise were anti-rickets factors. Later work would show that, in a way, everyone was correct. Puppies eating a poor diet, but playing outside, did develop strong bones. However, it was the exposure to sun, not the exercise, that strengthened the young canine skeleton.

Post–World War I Investigations into Rickets in Berlin, Vienna, and New York

More opportunities to investigate rickets came after World War I, when there was much malnutrition in Europe and many orphans. Orphans were placed in institutions. This social tragedy had the unexpected effect of making childhood illnesses more obvious and experiments easier to organize. A German physician, Kurt Huldschinsky, aware of the beliefs that cod-liver oil and sunshine prevented rickets, performed an amazing experiment in Berlin with babies with rickets. He had no access to cod-liver oil in those difficult postwar years, and sunshine in Germany did not seem strong enough to be beneficial. In 1919 he learned about the newly manufactured mercury vapor lamp:

> [Huldschinsky] picked out four of the most fidgety, pain-racked, and feeble rickety babies . . . and he did nothing at all to them but bathe their backs and sick pot-bellies in a violet bath of a sun-lamp's light . . . Was the virtue of the sun's rays there? Nobody knew . . . Huldschinsky set up his electric lamp, whose strange flame burned in an atmosphere of the vapor of mercury. Its light was an outlandish violet that hid in it burning, searing, powerful invisible rays that were beyond the violet . . . His rickety, wretched, continually crying and puling babies, Huldschinsky rayed the first day for just one minute, with the lamp not too close to their backs and bellies. Then five, then ten, then fifteen, then twenty minutes . . . They smiled . . . Two months of the eerie light of the lamp: they were strong. . . .[2]

In this vivid description of Huldschinsky's work, the author has graphically but misleadingly described the process. The light coming from the mercury vapor lamps may have looked violet, but the radiation that was so helpful was ultraviolet radiation, which is invisible. Huldschinksy's experiment was groundbreaking.

Malnutrition was rife in postwar Vienna and milk, butter, and eggs were scarce. The Lister Institute in London sent Harriette Chick to Vienna in 1922 to assist in the feeding of starving Viennese children. (Chick, formerly a bacteriologist, had made important discoveries with respect to Vitamin C just a few years earlier. She must have realized that her days of bacteriology had ended.) Chick had to overcome the distrust and skepticism of the Viennese. She impressed them by curing one child's scurvy with lemon juice and one child's eye ulcer with butterfat. Having won over her foreign colleagues, she proceeded to study the orphans, many ill with multiple diseases, including scurvy and tuberculosis. Her work was similar to that done by Goldberger in the orphanages in the southern United States. She controlled the diet of babies—known as foundlings—in Viennese orphanages. She and her colleagues divided the foundlings into groups and in a number of different experiments tried treatment with cod-liver oil, sunshine, or Huldschinsky's mercury vapor lamp. She used X-rays to confirm the diagnosis of rickets in these children and document their recovery. She confirmed all of the previous anecdotal observations and experience of clinicians:

- Toddlers were particularly prone to developing this illness.
- Sunshine and cod-liver oil prevented and cured rickets.
- Huldschinsky's mercury vapor lamp cured rickets.
- Rickets was worse in the winter.
- Fresh air and exercise did not prevent or treat rickets.

Some aspects of her work illustrate the differences with research in the twenty-first century. As we have seen in previous chapters, there seems to have been little oversight or concern about informed consent or the "use" of such vulnerable people. The use of X-rays, in retrospect, seems unfortunate, given what we now know about their dangers. These caveats aside, Chick was a careful scientist, and her work established definitively the roles of sunlight and cod-liver oil in treating and preventing rickets.

Work was also being done in New York. Alfred Hess (1875–1933) was a pediatrician working in New York. He attended Columbia and Harvard and trained in medicine at the College of Physicians and Surgeons in New York City. He studied in Berlin, Prague, and Vienna. He returned to New York and became a practicing clinician. In a previous chapter, we reviewed his observations about scurvy in infants. He was similar to some other researchers, such as R. R. Williams, Goldberger, or Sommer—all of whom made epidemiological and or laboratory findings with respect to vitamins and also organized or pioneered public health campaigns to address the deficiencies. Rickets was very common in his patients, especially dark-skinned babies. He organized a six-month trial of daily cod-liver oil for sixty-five infants. The cod-liver oil prevented the development of rickets; untreated babies developed the disease. He established a rickets clinic in 1917.

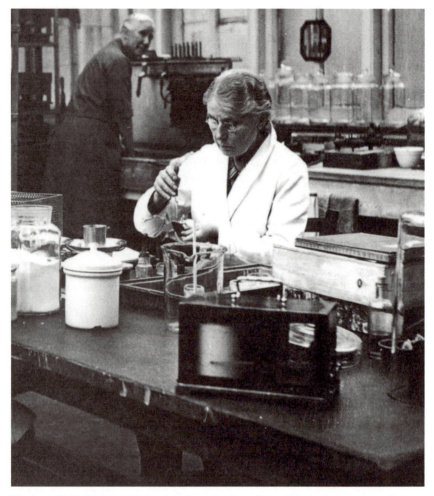

Harriette Chick (1875–1977), originally trained as a bacteriologist, became one of
the most prominent nutritional scientists of the twentieth century, and made contributions
to understanding Vitamin C and D. She is shown here in the conservatory animal house
at Roebuck House in Cambridge. She did much work at the Lister Institute in London,
but many animals and workers were evacuated to Cambridge during World War II.
Wellcome Library, London.

In 1921 Hess repeated Huldschinsky's trials and found that mercury
vapor quartz lamps and/or sunlight helped rickety rats and rickety children.
In 1923 Hess and Mildred Weinstock experimented with mercury vapor
lamps, filters, and rats to characterize the radiation. The anti-rickets radiation
proved to be in a narrow band of radiation, with a wavelength not longer
than about 300 nm and was, therefore, invisible because visible light has a
longer wavelength of 400–700 nm.

Mellanby Visits the Hebrides

Mellanby, in addition to working with puppies, also studied the diets of people throughout the United Kingdom. From 1920 to 1922 he described nutritional and general living conditions in the Hebrides, a chain of islands off the west coast of Scotland. The Hebrides was poor, and the people lived in primitive conditions. Heat came from peat fires. Houses had no windows and were dark and smoky. Babies were rarely taken outside. The conditions seemed certain to cause ill health. Once again, as shown by Palm, dirt and poor hygiene did not necessarily lead to rickets. Palm had emphasized the importance of sunlight, but these toddlers never saw the sun. It did not matter because the diet of the Hebrideans made up for the dirt and gloom. These children were breastfed and, after being weaned, consumed the regular adult Hebridean diet, which consisted of codheads stuffed with cod liver, milk, other fish, turnips, oatmeal, and potatoes. Thanks to this extraordinary diet, the children flourished, and rickets was never seen.

COD-LIVER OIL

Cod is a lean fish but has oil in its liver. Although cod-liver oil is famous for its Vitamin D content, many other fish actually have higher Vitamin D concentrations. However, cod, more than other fish, is prolific. Cod was the main fish in northern waters until recent overfishing. Cod-liver oil was used for hundreds of years by people who lived along the coast of northern oceans for its beneficial effects. They both ate it and rubbed it into their skin. Cod-liver oil is also high in Vitamin A.

The investigations of Chick, Mellanby, Huldschinsky, and Hess made it clear that rickets could be prevented or treated by sunlight, mercury vapor quartz lamps, cod-liver oil, and perhaps butterfat. However, the actual cause of rickets was not understood.

Work in Wisconsin and Baltimore—Heating and Aerating Cod-Liver Oil and the Discovery of Vitamin D

McCollum and his group, now famous for their discovery of Vitamin A, had moved to Johns Hopkins in Baltimore in 1917. A Johns Hopkins pediatrician, Howland, asked McCollum if he had produced rickets experimentally in his rats. He had. This was the beginning of a fruitful collaboration. Howland and other physicians at Hopkins were experts in histology, the microscopic study of tissues. They were able to see that, through the lens of the microscope, rickets in children was very similar to experimental rickets in rats. Narrowing down the actual deficiency in the diet that caused rickets in the rats was difficult. It seemed to be related to animal fats. Once again, as with the work with Vitamin A, the work was challenging. The diets had to be palatable and complete in everything except the rickets-preventing factor. The diets had to contain suitable amounts of the minerals needed to mineralize the bones, such as calcium and phosphorus. The diets had to keep the rats alive long enough to develop rickets. Rats that died too young never had the opportunity to develop rickets. The diet had to be better tasting than the rats themselves. Otherwise, the rats attacked, killed, and ate the weakest, which complicated the analyses of the diet.

McCollum formulated many diets. Diet number 3143 turned out to be the key diet for determining the causes of rickets. Rats grew well on 3143, did not resort to cannibalism, but did become rickety. Cod-liver oil added to the diet prevented rickets. Butterfat was less helpful. McCollum and his group concluded that a fat-soluble substance was missing from 3143. Butterfat and cod-liver oil contain Vitamin A. Was Vitamin A deficiency the cause of rickets? In Cambridge, Hopkins had earlier shown that Vitamin A was inactivated by heating or bubbling air through cod-liver oil. McCollum did just this to cod-liver oil and found the oil still could prevent rickets. There was a substance in cod-liver oil that withstood heating and exposure to air and, therefore, was not Vitamin A. This substance was the anti-rickets factor and was named Vitamin D in 1922.

Rickets—One Disease, Two Cures, and the Mysterious Jars

McCollum also took rats into the sun. Rats fed diet 3143 and exposed to the sun did not become rickety. This was peculiar. Diet 3143 supported life and growth, but without Vitamin D or sunlight, it led to rickets. It seemed that rickets was one disease with two cures. Was there any connection between the sunlight and the newly discovered Vitamin D? Another University of Wisconsin scientist was one of the researchers who worked out the connection.

Harry Steenbock (1886–1967) grew up on a family farm in Wisconsin. He worked with Babcock and McCollum and then himself became a researcher at the University of Wisconsin. Steenbock was aware of strange findings from England, where scientists had continued Huldschinsky's work. They confirmed his success with children by going back to the laboratory. They irradiated rats and cured their rickets. The English scientists extended these observations. Ill rats were placed in the jars that had been irradiated and became well. It was as though the air could be irradiated, hold on to the radiation, and cure the rats. Steenbock repeated these experiments and made even more curious observations. Rickety rats were exposed to healthy irradiated rats and became healthier. Originally, it was thought that the irradiated rats might themselves be emitting ultraviolet rays. This was an ingenious idea. In some unusual circumstances, organisms can become "radioactive," but that only happens with quite different types of radiation. Mercury vapor lamps emit ultraviolet radiation that is not "radioactive" in the sense of leading to organisms emitting radiation.

Observations continued. Even if the ill rats were put in cages which had housed the well rats previously, this was enough to improve their health. It turned out that the jars were not, in fact, empty. They contained sawdust bedding that had inadvertently been irradiated. Steenbock irradiated cages with only screens in them, so that all of the bedding could be removed. Ill rats were moved into these cages in which there had been well rats and no bedding. Even in these empty cages, the health of the rats improved. After many more experiments, including ones in which cages were placed on top of one another, Steenbock concluded that the screens themselves were sometimes soiled with rat feces and that the rats would then consume the feces on the screens or that had dropped down from the other cages. The health-giving "contagious" factor was due to:

- Ill rats eating bedding that had developed Vitamin D after being irradiated.
- Ill rats eating the droppings of healthy rats, which contained Vitamin D.
- Ill rats licking their paws, which had picked up Vitamin D from rat feces smeared onto the screens in the cages.

(Feces also contains Vitamin A, B9, and B12.)

Eventually, these experiments and observations led to an understanding of this odd vitamin. By the early 1920s, Steenbock knew that irradiating rodent food chow prevented the rats from developing rickets. Radiation of the sterols in the food, including the food that had spilled into the sawdust, led to the formation of Vitamin D. Steenbock went back to McCollum's famous diet 3143. This time, he did not add any fats to it. Instead, he irradiated it and discovered that the irradiated diet could cure rickets.

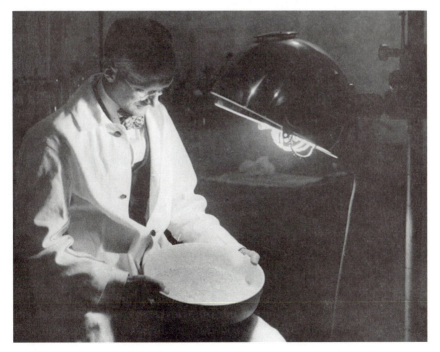

Harry Steenbock (1886–1967) is radiating unknown material to form Vitamin D. Picture is from about 1929. Courtesy University of Wisconsin–Madison Archives.

Patenting Irradiation and Protecting the Dairy Industry

Steenbock decided that he did not want his irradiation discovery to have the same fate as Babcock's test for determining the butterfat content of milk. He was intent on keeping control of the process to protect the public from flawed preparations. In 1924, he spent three hundred dollars to file a patent application. Meanwhile, Quaker Oats realized the marketing opportunities that would have flowed from their ability to offer cereal fortified with Vitamin D. Because of the work of Mellanby, oatmeal had developed a bad reputation of being associated with rickets. Quaker wanted to establish oatmeal as a healthy food. Quaker offered Steenbock nearly a million dollars for rights to his discovery or patent. Steenbock turned Quaker down. Steenbock approached administrators at the University of Wisconsin in Madison with the suggestion that the university establish an agency to protect discoveries made by the faculty, bringing profits back to the university to manage the financial and administrative tasks that came with patents.

Steenbock's decision to patent this discovery through the university was controversial. (R. R. Williams' decision to patent the steps in his synthesis of thiamine would cause him some trouble a few years later.) Was it ethical to patent such an important discovery? The University of Wisconsin is a land grant university, meaning that it was publicly funded. Therefore, some people thought that the discovery should not be patented but rather that it should be given to the public. The university was initially quite apprehensive, but, eventually, much to its future profit, it agreed to take a role in patenting Steenbock's process. In November of 1925, at a cost of nine hundred dollars, the Wisconsin Alumni Research Foundation (WARF) was established. It became a wealthy and important "technology transfer" foundation. In 1928, Steenbock obtained his patent.

Most of WARF's income comes from Vitamin D. As of 2007, WARF has given over nine hundred million dollars back to the University of Wisconsin to fund more research. This excellent return on twelve hundred dollars (Steenbock's original three hundred dollar patent application plus the nine hundred dollars that the university paid to establish WARF) has been noticed. Many other universities now hold patents for discoveries made by their faculty members and make healthy profits.

WARF AND WARFARIN

The discovery of coumadin took place at the University of Wisconsin. A Wisconsin farmer saw cows bleed to death after eating spoiled sweet clover hay. This substance, coumadin, was developed by the university and subsequently used as a rodenticide. Coumadin is now also used as a medication to prevent dangerous blood clots in humans. This substance was patented under the name "warfarin."

WARF sold the rights to a number of companies (including Quaker Oats), allowing them to add Vitamin D to substances, such as breakfast cereals. One of the most difficult food products to enrich with Vitamin D was milk. Pure food laws at the time prevented milk from being supplemented with any product. So, odd as it seems now, the milk itself was irradiated. (Nowadays, milk is no longer irradiated. Vitamin D is added to milk.)

Steenbock had another motive in protecting his invention. Like his University of Wisconsin predecessors Babcock and McCollum, Steenbock was protective of the dairy farmers. He did not want margarine manufacturers fortifying their artificial product with Vitamin D and then touting its equivalence—or perhaps even superiority—over natural butter. McCollum had been opposed to vitamin supplementation of all foods. Steenbock did not carry this attitude as far as did McCollum, but he continued in the Wisconsin tradition of protecting "sweet" butter against the "abomination" of margarine by blocking, for as long as he could, the supplementation of margarine with Vitamin A.

In 1924 Hess in New York independently showed that ultraviolet irradiation of foods gave them anti-rickets properties. The work of Hess and Steenbock meant that within a few years, children in the United States were eating irradiated bread, and milk and rickets (almost) disappeared.

Vitamin D: More Surprises and More Patents

Hess and others had suspected that cholesterol, a sterol in the skin, might be the substance that was converted into an anti-rickets agent by ultraviolet light. To investigate this, he invited Adolf Windaus (1876–1959), the world's leading expert in sterols, to come to New York. In the early 1900s, sterols in cell membranes interested few people. Windaus, a German organic chemist, learned everything that he could about these molecules, trusting that at some time they would prove to be interesting. Hess and Windaus collaborated with a team led by Otto Rosenheim in London. These men worked together amicably and in 1926 showed that cholesterol was not the anti-rickets substance. A molecule related to cholesterol, ergosterol, a fungal sterol, when irradiated, became Vitamin D2 or calciferol. Windaus was awarded the Nobel Prize in 1928 for his work with sterols. This was the first Nobel Prize to be awarded that was associated with Vitamin D, or indeed with any vitamin. However, ergosterol was only found in plants and fungi. In the mid-1930s, Windaus studied 7-dehydrocholesterol, another relative of cholesterol, found in animals, and showed that this molecule was changed by radiation into Vitamin D3 or cholecalciferol.

More work in the second half of the twentieth century explained how the vitamin works and revealed some of the complexities. With the use of radioisotopes, the vitamin was able to be followed closely in the body. Much of this work was done by Hector DeLuca and colleagues at the University of Wisconsin. DeLuca was the last student of Steenbock. When Steenbock retired in 1955, DeLuca took over his laboratory, and he has spent his career working with Vitamin D.

In 1968 Hector DeLuca and his colleagues at Wisconsin showed that the formation of active Vitamin D requires more than sunlight and involves more organs than just the skin. Once formed in the skin, Vitamin D has to be changed in the liver to a slightly different form of the molecule. Michael F. Holick at Wisconsin was a student of DeLuca's. He is yet another link in the chain of University of Wisconsin vitamin researchers. Holick and DeLuca, and Andrew W. Norman in California and Egon Kodicek in Cambridge, England, showed that the form of Vitamin D from the liver also had to be changed in the kidney before it could become the biologically active form of the vitamin—calcitriol. This was yet another surprise. Until that point, the kidney had been thought of primarily as the organ that filters the blood and "cleans" it by making urine. The kidney turned out to be an organ closely involved, because of its work with Vitamin D, with the health of the body's bones. Holick, then working in Boston, later demonstrated the exact steps by which ultraviolet B radiation changed 7-dehydrocholesterol in the skin into Vitamin D3.

Vitamin D: A Hormone

Vitamin D, similar to retinoic acid, a Vitamin A molecule, is active within the nucleus of the cell, where it interacts with the gene to change enzyme production. Active Vitamin D, or calcitriol, leads to more transport proteins in the intestines, which increases calcium absorption. Like other hormones, Vitamin D is subject to feedback. If dietary calcium is high, Vitamin D levels decrease, and if blood calcium levels drop, Vitamin D will "take" calcium from the bone. Vitamin D works in concert with other hormones, particularly parathyroid hormone, to regulate the complicated relationships between calcium in the bone and blood.

Vitamin D: Not Just Skin and Bone

Now at Boston University, Holick and others showed that the active form of the vitamin can also be produced in other cells of the body, such as breast, colon, and prostate. Vitamin D controls over two hundred genes that are active in the immune response to infections and cancer cells. Holick and others have shown that Vitamin D has many more effects in the body than had been understood previously, including fighting autoimmune illnesses, heart disease, and some cancers. Cells throughout the body "recognize" Vitamin D.

A Resurgence of Rickets

The avoidance of sunshine, for fear of wrinkles or skin cancer, leads to Vitamin D deficiency. This risk is particularly severe in people who:

- Live far from the equator, wear clothes covering most of the body, or use sunscreen.
- Are old, because synthesis of 7-dehydrocholesterol decreases with age.
- Are obese, because Vitamin D is trapped in fat cells.

- Are ill with liver or kidney failure.
- Take certain medications, such as antiseizure or anti-AIDS medication.
- Are dark skinned, because melanin is a sunscreen.

Rickets is again becoming more common, especially in dark-skinned children living in climates where they are not exposed to the sun or in children of any pigmentation who are protected from the sun. Without sufficient Vitamin D, adults develop osteomalacia and muscle weakness and are at increased risk of multiple other chronic illnesses, including some cancers, multiple sclerosis, and cardiovascular illness.

Moderate exposure to the ultraviolet B radiation of sunshine is currently recommended by Vitamin D experts. This is controversial because many dermatologists recommend avoidance of the sun. With most other vitamins, deficiency can be avoided by a sensible diet, but Vitamin D is not contained in many foods, and few people, other than those of northern European fishing communities and the Hebrides, enjoy the taste of cod-liver oil. Vitamin D experts recommend Vitamin D supplementation in the absence of sun exposure.

SUMMARY

Rickets captured the imagination of many chroniclers of the eighteenth and nineteenth centuries. Children who could not bear their own weight without bending their legs into curves formed a vivid picture. The cause of this was a lack of a vitamin that is not a vitamin. Sunshine on our skin is all we need. McCollum, Steenbock, Hess, Chick, and others showed that rats and rickety children grow strong bones with the aid of sunshine, ultraviolet B radiation, or cod-liver oil. The solar radiation, which is so important for our health, occupies a small band of the solar radiation reaching the Earth. Solar radiation consists of radiation, with a wavelength of 100–700 nm. Visible light has a wavelength of 400–700 nm. The ultraviolet B radiation that activates 7-dehydrocholesterol is only that between 290 and 315 nm.

In other chapters, vitamin deficiencies have been described mostly as diseases of adventurers, such as scurvy, or of the poor, such as Vitamin A deficiency, or of those with autoimmune illnesses, such as pernicious anemia. These disorders are, for the most part, very rare in the developed world. Vitamin D deficiency, in contrast, is widespread in the developed world and is becoming more common. The discovery of Vitamin D was to do with rickets, but, in Holick's words, rickets is only the "tip of the Vitamin D-deficiency iceberg."[3]

7

CAN YOU HAVE TOO MUCH OF A GOOD THING? TOXICITY FROM VITAMINS

Vitamins A and D are stored in the liver and fat cells. This means that these vitamins do not have to be taken on a daily basis, but the downside is that large doses of these vitamins can be stored in the body. Toxicity from the fat-soluble vitamins is unusual but serious. Large doses of water-soluble vitamins are usually excreted in the urine and cause little damage. Once again, the intrepid explorers of the poles helped to demonstrate some truths about vitamins. Vitamin deficiencies occurred in the midst of many other deprivations; vitamin toxicity also sometimes happened.

EXCESSIVE CONSUMPTION: THE FRANKLIN EXPEDITION REDUX

Eating liver is generally safe in moderation, but there were circumstances in the past in which consumption of large quantities of liver caused hypervitaminosis A. This happened to some explorers of the Arctic and Antarctic. Vitamin A toxicity became widely appreciated as a result of the tumult around the Franklin Expedition, described earlier in this book. Although an English catastrophe, the complete disappearance of this well-supplied expedition attracted worldwide notice and dominated headlines across the Atlantic. One person who followed it closely was Elisha Kent Kane (1820–1857), an American physician. Kane participated in two searches for Franklin. He was a naval surgeon with one expedition in 1850–1851 and led his own expedition two years later.

Kane's expedition lasted from 1853–1855 and was unsuccessful. In August 1854, half of his crew defected, only to return several months later, frostbitten and starving. Without the help of the Inuit (the Eskimo people), they would have died. Kane's lengthy and detailed account of this expedition became a best seller. He spent nine hundred pages describing the frigid hell of Arctic travel. This was at a time when the reading public had no movies or television, so people had a high tolerance of long books, and, as noted before, one of life's strange pleasures is reading of the misfortunes of others.

Kane was one of the first explorers to realize that the Inuit had much knowledge to impart to others about how to survive in the Arctic. The Inuit had a diet that is quite different from the Western diet. They ate large quantities of fish and seal. An important part of their diet was liver from various animals. (The Inuit had low rates of cardiovascular illness in the past, when they were physically active and followed this diet.) They knew that they had to be careful about the liver that they ate. They knew that polar bear liver—which is richer in Vitamin A than the liver of other animals—was dangerous, and they avoided it.

Kane was a good student and observer. Unlike many other explorers, he was ready to learn from the indigenous people. Kane learned from the Inuit the dangers of eating polar bear liver. In 1856 he wrote about the neurological side effects that come from eating too much of this type of liver. He described vertigo, headache, drowsiness, and irritability. Kane's best seller contained the first widely read description of Vitamin A toxicity.

A Snow Bridge Collapses; Man's Best Friend Disappoints

Vitamin A toxicity was also described at the other end of the world. Explorers of the Antarctic experienced all the difficulties that their northern colleagues did, and more. Travel in the Antarctic was worse than in the Arctic because of the extreme cold and high winds. The winds form long, wave-like ridges of snow known as sastrugi, which hinder travel. Sastrugi are not found in the Arctic. Deep fissures or cracks in the packed snow or ice, known as crevasses, were common, and often difficult to see.

In 1911, Douglas Mawson (1882–1958) led an expedition to map and explore the coastal area of Antarctica. He took with him a small team of men, including the Swiss scientist Dr. Xavier Mertz (1883–1912) and Lieutenant Belgrave Ninnis (?–1912). Nineteen Greenland huskies pulled the expedition's sleds. On November 10, 1912, Mawson, Mertz, and Ninnis set out to explore the coast. On December 13, they cautiously divided up their supplies into two sleds and put the more important supplies into the second sled, thinking that if any sled would disappear into an unseen crevasse, it would be the first sled. On December 14, Mertz was skiing ahead of the other two. He sang as he skied. Mawson was traveling in the first sled, and he was followed by Ninnis, with the important second sled. Mertz stopped singing and signaled that he was crossing a snow bridge over a crevasse. Mawson's sledge passed over the crevasse uneventfully; in turn, he signaled its presence to Ninnis. However, Mertz on his skis and then Mawson's sledge must have weakened the snow bridge over the crevasse. Ninnis and the second sled broke through the bridge and fell into the crevasse. They disappeared. Mawson and Mertz turned back but could find no trace of them in the crevasse, which was over one hundred fifty feet deep. Ninnis, the second sled, most of the supplies, and many of the huskies had disappeared forever.

Mertz and Mawson were left with very little food. The two men ate the huskies one by one. Their flesh was difficult to chew, particularly as the men were beginning to lose their teeth from scurvy. The easiest part of the dog to eat was the large tender liver. Mertz became increasingly ill. Mawson gave him most of the dog liver to eat, in part because of its tenderness. Mertz worsened. He blamed it on the dog diet. His skin began to peel off. He became uncharacteristically irritable and morose. He complained of terrible headaches. He became confused, delirious, and violent. He died on January 7, 1913.[1]

Mertz's sense that his dog diet was not good for him was correct. His miseries were caused in part by Vitamin A toxicity. Husky liver is similar to polar bear liver in that it is rich in Vitamin A. Mawson worsened Mertz's misery by preferentially giving him the canine livers. Kane had written of the dangers of polar bear liver; and Mawson and Mertz had demonstrated the dangers of husky liver.

HYPERVITAMINOSIS A

Some people take large doses of Vitamin A hoping for improved vision, increased resistance to disease, improved skin, and the like. The result is often a condition marked by dry skin, vomiting, hair loss, bone pain, and irritability. There is a particular danger for women. If a pregnant woman consumes large amounts of Vitamin A, she is at risk for miscarriages or giving birth to a baby with malformations. Too much Vitamin A may also be harmful for bones, especially those of old people.[2]

CAN CARROTS MAKE YOU MAD?

It is difficult to develop Vitamin A toxicity from eating too many carotenoids because they are not converted to the active vitamin at a very high rate. Carotenoids do have the effect of giving some vegetables, such as carrots, and some animals their typical orange color. Pink flamingos, red salmon, and red lobsters owe their color to these carotenoids. People who eat carrots with abandon can develop a yellow or orange discoloration to their skin. Apart from the possible embarrassment caused by their resemblance to flamingos, salmon, or lobsters, the condition is not harmful.

IS TREATMENT FOR ACNE SAFE?

A syndrome resembling Vitamin A toxicity may occur in some people who take the antiacne medication, isotretinoin. Isotretinoin (also known as Accutane®) is a member of the retinoid family of drugs, which are derivatives of Vitamin A or retinol. Accutane® was synthesized in 1955 and has been used for the treatment of acne since 1971. Because isotretinoin is a relative of Vitamin A, many of the side effects seen with isotretinoin are similar to those seen in hypervitaminosis A. Isotretinoin is particularly dangerous to pregnant women because of the risks to the fetus. Some physicians and researchers have also suggested that isotretinoin may be linked to depression and suicide and have even found some changes in brain function in people taking this medication.[3]

HYPERVITAMINOSIS D: EUROPE IN THE 1950s

Many infants in Europe in the past suffered from rickets. Therefore, when Vitamin D was discovered, it was only natural that Vitamin D was administered to children to prevent this disfiguring disease. In the 1950s many infants developed high calcium levels, thought to be due to overly generous Vitamin D supplementation. Children suffered loss of appetite, vomiting, constipation, confusion, slowed growth, listlessness, calcium deposits in the kidney, and sometimes death. Some European governments banned Vitamin D fortification of milk because of this.[4] Occasional cases of hypervitaminosis D continue to be reported. This is due, oddly, to the cheapness of the vitamin. Because it is so cheap, people are sometimes careless in how much is put into milk or supplements. People with certain illnesses may be particularly sensitive to Vitamin D. Sun exposure will not lead to Vitamin D toxicity. This is because solar radiation leads to Vitamin D3 but also leads to its breakdown. Also, exposure to sun stimulates the production of the pigment melanin, which acts as a sunscreen.

8

CONCLUSION: VICTORIES, BUT LINGERING CONCERNS

The scientists who discovered vitamins changed how we understood nutrition, the causes of some illnesses, and how our bodies work. It is clear to us now, after the brilliant work of McCollum, Funk, and Hopkins, among others, that we need "ready-made" compounds, which are the vitamins—but this was far from obvious before the work of these scientists that was described in this book.

In telling these stories, several themes have emerged. For example, we saw that there was an ongoing conflict between physicians who saw illnesses as caused by microorganisms and physicians who saw illnesses as caused by a dietary deficiency. Louis Pasteur in France and Robert Koch in Germany made astonishing discoveries about microbes and their ability to cause illnesses in the late 1800s. Physicians wondered if all illnesses would turn out to be caused by bacteria and other microbes. However, bacteria, in addition to being harmful, produce vitamins (for example, cobalamin), which, in very small amounts, are essential parts of our diet. Plants, although they are immobile, insensate, and without any central nervous system, also have intracellular machinery capable of making pro–Vitamin A (carotenoids). We depend on these simpler organisms for our health. The discovery of vitamins—even smaller than microorganisms—depended on the ability of other scientists to look beyond the important contributions of Pasteur and Koch and understand that illnesses could be related to diet.

Yet another theme is how diseases and the discovery of vitamins often depended on seemingly unconnected technological advances. For example, the invention of steam-powered rollers in the 1800s made the milling of rice much easier; this, in turn, increased the incidence of beriberi, which eventually led to the discovery of thiamine. Improvements in navigation skills led to long sea voyages, which led to scurvy. The invention and development of computers helped to make Dorothy Hodgkin's characterization of the complicated cobalamin molecule possible.

Many of the scientists performed experiments that are shocking to us today. Scientists and physicians performed experiments on prisoners, orphans, patients in asylums, and others, never thinking to get their permission. Standards have changed, yet these experiments, much as they would be disapproved of now, were important in leading to discoveries that were immensely helpful to the health of many.

Finally, these discoveries were important for more reasons than nutrition. The discovery of Vitamin A has led to insights in vision, cell growth, and immunity from illnesses. Explorations into Vitamin C have clarified the structure of collagen and cartilage, the materials that hold us together. The scientists who studied Vitamin D have helped to explain more of the mysteries surrounding the regulation of cell growth.

Much work remains to be done. Vitamin D deficiency may be widespread in the United States and other developed countries. Vitamin A deficiency is a common cause of blindness and mortality in the developing world. Many of the scientists in this book, such as Aykroyd, Williams, and Goldberger, noted the connections between poverty and malnutrition. Those connections still exist. Chapters about how to ensure that all people, no matter where they live, have access to healthy diets, so that all of humanity can benefit from the discoveries described in this book, remain to be written.

Appendix A

Vitamin A and the Eye

Vitamin A, Rods and Cones, and Rhodopsin

Rods and cones in the retina, the back of eye, are photoreceptor cells. Light striking these cells is responsible for our vision. Rods are far more sensitive to light than the cones, but they do not differentiate between colors. Therefore, during the day, at high light levels, the rods are "bleached out," and we use our cones and see colors. At dawn or dusk, the rods take over, and we can see, but only in black and white.

In the retina, Vitamin A is converted into retinal. Retinal combines with opsin in the retina to form rhodopsin, also known as visual purple. Rhodopsin is contained in the rods and is needed for vision in dim light. When light hits rhodopsin, the structure of retinal changes and sends a message to the brain that there is something seen. Animals that hunt at night, such as lions and owls, have eyes with high numbers of rods and dense concentrations of visual purple.

Vitamin A, Night Blindness, and Xerophthalmia

Night blindness or the inability to see in dim light is due to insufficient retinal in the rods of the eye. Night blindness is difficult to recognize in children until they are walking independently. At that time, parents or others will notice the toddler bumping and falling as the light fades.

Xerophthalmia means dry eye. It is the leading cause of acquired blindness in children in the world. It is often preceded by night blindness and can be irreversible if not treated early. Without Vitamin A the glands of the eyes, which produce tears to protect the eye, stop producing this fluid and the conjunctiva, the thin, clear membrane over the white of the eye, becomes dry. The cornea, the transparent dome over the center of the eye that protects the pupil and also acts as a lens, becomes inflamed or infected. Then, ulcers and scars develop on the cornea, eventually leading to corneal destruction resulting in permanent blindness.

Can Extra Vitamin A Improve One's Night Vision?

The British Air Force wanted the Nazis to think so in World War II. In the early 1940s, British pilots were performing well, and the British circulated the story that this was due to the pilots eating carrots. This was widely believed but not true. This was British propaganda, designed to fool the Germans. The British pilots were doing well because of the improved radar. It was to the advantage of the British military that the German military worry about the vegetables that the pilots were eating rather than the radar that they were using.

Appendix B

CALCIUM, BONES, AND COLLAGEN

CALCIUM

Calcium is the most abundant metal in the human body. The average male adult body contains about 1200 g of calcium. Most of this calcium is located in bones as calcium phosphate. The discovery of Vitamin D was due to its role in increasing absorption of calcium and phosphorus from food in the gastrointestinal tract. Without enough Vitamin D, bones have insufficient calcium and become soft. The remaining portion of the body's calcium (as little as about 10 g) is in the blood. This calcium is essential for the smooth operation of many of the body's tasks, such as normal nerve and muscle action.

CALCIUM AS A BUILDING STRUCTURE

Humans use calcium to form a hard skeleton. Calcium also is used in many other structures because, in combination with other elements, it forms hard substances that retain their shape and can withstand pressure and exposure to water and wind.

Other organisms build objects with calcium. Corals, small soft-bodied animals, secrete calcium carbonate to make some of the largest structures in the world— coral reefs. Calcium, in various forms, is a structural component in many structures in the inanimate world. Limestone is calcium carbonate. It is a commonly mined rock and a key component of many buildings. Cement, composed of limestone, silica, and iron, is used to bind building materials together. Mixed with water and sand, cement becomes concrete, a common building material. Mixed with lime, cement becomes mortar, another agent used to hold building materials together. Hydrated calcium sulfate is known as gypsum, which makes up plasterboard and plaster of Paris.

BONES

The 206 bones in the human adult form the skeleton and are responsible for the shape of the body and the protection of the soft and vulnerable tissues and organs. The skeleton is often compared with the girders and beams of buildings (or vice versa), but bone faces more challenges than does the skeleton of buildings. Bone has to grow and support movement. It also stores and releases calcium and provides a home for stem cells.

As the body develops, bone has to become bigger, but this must be regulated very carefully because the bone must always be proportional to other organs. In addition to growing during childhood and adolescence, bone can change during adulthood. Bone that is stressed by being pulled on or tugged at or bearing weight loads will actually become more dense. Bones are involved in movement of the body. Without the stabilizing and leveraging presence of bones, movement would be very different. Bones also must withstand immense pressure when the body moves; for example, when we run or move objects. Special cells, known as osteoblasts and osteoclasts, are constantly changing bone. Osteoblasts make collagen and lay down calcium phosphate to form new bone. Osteoclasts break down bone so that bone can be remodeled.

Calcium moves in and out of bone. If necessary, bone will release calcium to ensure adequate blood levels of calcium. Bone hardness is sacrificed to the overall welfare of the electrical system of the body, particularly the conduction system of the heart. Therefore, bones are a reservoir of calcium or a safety net and a structural component of the body. Vitamin D and other hormones are involved in the building and maintenance of bone while at the same time maintaining a steady calcium level in blood. Finally, bone contains bone marrow. This soft and fatty tissue is found in the hollow interior of some of the body's larger bones. Stem cells in marrow produce the body's blood cells.

COLLAGEN

Collagen, the most common protein in the body, is an important part of the skin, tendons, ligaments, scar tissue, blood vessel walls, and bone. Ascorbic acid, or Vitamin C, is needed for the activity of the enzymes that synthesize collagen. Collagen is formed by three strands of amino acids. Two strands are coiled into a left-handed triple helix. Three of these coils weave themselves into a right-handed cable, known as a super helix or coiled coil. This super helix has more strength for its weight than steel. Collagen is responsible for bone's flexibility and resilience. Calcium and phosphorus coat the collagen, or mineralize it, in the matrix of the bone to make it hard.

Without adequate Vitamin C, collagen is not properly formed. Capillaries throughout the body leak, gums become swollen, wounds cannot heal, and bone is not correctly fashioned.

Appendix C

ANEMIA

There are more red blood cells than any other type of cell, and they make up half of the volume of our blood. Each cubic milliliter of blood contains about five million red blood cells. The cells are flattish disks with a "biconcave" shape. Red cells are produced in the bone marrow. Each red blood cell carries nearly three hundred million hemoglobin molecules. Hemoglobin is a complicated protein made up of heme, which contains four iron atoms, and globin. Each iron atom can carry one molecule of oxygen. Hemoglobin carries oxygen from the lungs to the rest of the body. When carrying oxygen, hemoglobin is red, which gives blood its distinctive color.

Oxygen is needed by the body's cells for energy. The cells "burn" glucose for energy and, in most cases, need oxygen to do this. Red blood cells carry oxygen from the oxygen-rich air in the lungs to the oxygen-poor parts of the body. The red blood cells have to "know" when to pick up and when to deliver. This task is achieved by the intricate nature of the proteins of hemoglobin and the pattern of electrons around the iron atom. Hemoglobin changes its shape to attract and to release oxygen depending on the oxygen levels surrounding it.

Red blood cells fit into the capillaries, small blood vessels, to deliver oxygen throughout of the body. The capillary is smaller than the red blood cell. The red blood cell, unlike other cells in the body, has no nucleus in it. The red blood cell squeezes into the narrow capillaries to provide oxygen to all body cells.

After a few months of relentless traveling and squeezing through small vessels, the red blood cells wear out and are recycled in the liver and the spleen. The hemoglobin is scavenged from the cells, and the iron is carried back to the bone marrow to be used for new red cells. The rest of the heme is broken down into bilirubin. About three million red blood cells are recycled by the liver every second. Folate and cobalamin are required for production of new red blood cells in the bone marrow.

Without enough of these two vitamins, red cells do not develop properly. With too few red cells, the heart works "harder" to provide oxygen to the rest of the body. The heart beats faster and pumps greater volumes of blood. The heart may become weakened from the excessive work. In some of the anemias where there is an excessive destruction of red blood cells, bilirubin builds up, making the person look yellow or jaundiced. Common symptoms of anemia include:

- Trouble thinking
- Weakness or dizziness
- Numb or cold hands or feet
- Headache
- Pale skin, pale fingertips or lips or fingernail beds, or a yellowish color to the skin
- Fast heartbeat or palpitations
- Shortness of breath
- Chest pain.

In both vitamin deficiency anemias, the red cells in the circulation and bone marrow are larger than normal. Because of these unusually large cells, the anemias are called megaloblastic or macrocytic.

Appendix D

HOW MUCH OF EACH VITAMIN SHOULD I TAKE?

In 1941, the recommended daily allowances (RDAs) were established to answer the question: how much of each vitamin do we need? This was prompted in part by the need for food rationing during World War II. In 1997, a new term was developed: daily recommended intake (DRI). The answer became more involved, and the acronyms multiplied.

DRI is an overarching concept that includes the RDA, but also other quantities, known as the estimated average requirement (EAR), adequate intake (AI), and tolerable upper level (TUL). This proliferation of acronyms has been confusing. Agencies in other countries have different recommendations and different acronyms. This confusion reflects the difficulty in making exact recommendations. Each person's requirement for vitamins is somewhat different because it depends on many factors, such as:

- Stage of development
- Activity level
- Composition of diet
- Pregnancy
- Presence of any bowel diseases
- General state of health
- Alcohol intake
- Unknown metabolic differences between individuals.

Can we get any guidance from the scientists themselves? What diets did the protagonists of this book follow? Pauling attributed his ninety-three years to high doses of Vitamin C. He was unusual in his trust in vitamin megadoses. Chick lived past one hundred and was giving lectures well into her nineties. As far as is known, she did not give the credit to vitamins. McCollum lived until eighty-eight and was always outspoken in deriding the quackery and exploitation of the public by the vitamin pill sellers. Most of the scientists in this book who lived long lives did not worry about their own vitamin intake. Their health was due to other reasons: they ate diets with a variety of foods, did not indulge in excessive amounts of alcohol or nicotine, always looked before they crossed the street, had good genes, and, most important of all, were lucky.

Most people in the developed world who eat some animal products and fresh fruit and vegetables almost certainly have a diet containing enough vitamins and do not need to take multivitamins. Drinking vitamin-enriched water and sodas is helpful for the manufacturers of those products but not for the consumer. For some years, researchers had hoped that supplementation of diets with vitamins might prevent cancers, cardiovascular illnesses, or dementia, but the evidence from careful studies does not support this. Taking extra doses of vitamins is unlikely to prove to be the much-hunted-after elixir of youth. Vitamins are needed to prevent vitamin deficiency illnesses. There is not compelling evidence that taking high doses of vitamins can prolong our lives or compensate for eating too much, smoking, or not exercising.

There are two exceptions, one involving a vitamin and one involving groups of people. The vitamin exception is Vitamin D; experts in this area do believe that many in the developed world may be Vitamin D deficient because of limited exposure to the sun. The other exception is actually a group of exceptions. People with bowel diseases, the elderly, the pregnant, strict vegetarians, and those who take certain prescription medications or who abuse alcohol may need vitamin supplementation. As always, people should consult with their own physicians with respect to their own particular nutritional needs.

In summary, there is good evidence that people eating highly restricted diets become ill. There is little evidence that consuming high doses of vitamins can guarantee us youth and happiness. Would that it were otherwise.

NOTES

CHAPTER 1

1. E. V. McCollum, *From Kansas Farm Boy to Scientist* (Lawrence: University of Kansas Press, 1964), p. 114.

2. Ibid., p. 126.

3. E. V. McCollum and J. E. Becker, *Food, Nutrition, and Health*, 6th ed. (Baltimore, MD: The Lord Baltimore Press, 1947), p. 67.

4. G. Strey, "Wisconsin's Fight over the Demon Spread," *Wisconsin Magazine of History* (Autumn 2001): 3–15.

5. Ibid., pp. 5–6.

6. McCollum, p. 140.

7. Ibid., pp. 155–56.

8. A. Sommer, "A Bridge Too Near," in *The Progress of Nations* (New York: UNI-CEF, 1995), pp. 10–11.

CHAPTER 2

1. K. J. Carpenter, *Beriberi, White Rice, and Vitamin B. A Disease, a Cause, and a Cure* (Berkeley: University of California Press, 2000), p. 52.

2. Ibid., pp. 52–53.

3. Ibid., pp. 110–11.

4. A. Hardy, "Beriberi, Vitamin B1, and World Food Policy," *Medical History* 39 (1995): pp. 61–77.

5. Carpenter, pp. 171–72.

6. R. R. Williams, *Toward the Conquest of Beriberi* (Cambridge, MA: Harvard University Press, 1961), pp. 109–10.

7. R. C. Burgess, "Deficiency Diseases in Prisoners-of-War at Changi, Singapore," *Lancet* 2 (1946): 411–18.

8. Carpenter, p. 190.

9. L. R. Drew and A. S. Truswell, "Wernicke's Encephalopathy and Thiamine Fortification of Food: Time for a New Direction?" *Medical Journal of Australia* 168 (1998): 534–35.

10. M. Victor and P. I. Yakovlev, "S. S. Korsakoff's Psychic Disorder in Conjunction with Peripheral Neuritis. A Translation of Korsakoff's Original Article with Brief Comments on the Author and His Contributions to Clinical Medicine," *Neurology* 5 (1955): 394–406.

11. H. Klawans, *Newton's Madness. Further Tales of Clinical Neurology* (New York: Harper & Row, 1990), pp. 187–91.

CHAPTER 3

1. H. McGee, *On Food and Cooking: The Science and Lore of the Kitchen* (New York: Collier Books, Macmillan Publishing Company, 1984), p. 240.

2. E. W. Etheridge, *The Butterfly Caste: A Social History of Pellagra in the South* (Westport, CT: Greenwood, 1972), p. 9.

3. D. A. Roe, *A Plague of Corn. The Social History of Pellagra* (Ithaca, NY: Cornell University Press, 1973), pp. 37–38.

4. E. Fee, *Disease and Discovery. A History of the Johns Hopkins School of Hygiene and Public Health, 1916–1939* (Baltimore, MD: The Johns Hopkins University Press, 1987), p. 52.

5. Etheridge, p. 116.

6. M. F. Goldberger, "Dr. Joseph Goldberger—His Wife's Recollections," in A. M. Beeuwkes, E. N. Todhunter, and E. S. Weigley, eds. *Essays on History of Nutrition and Dietetics* (Chicago: The American Dietetic Association, 1967), pp. 284–87.

7. S. Lehrer, *Explorers of the Body* (New York: Doubleday & Company, Inc., 1979), pp. 360–61.

8. A. M. Kraut, *Goldberger's War: The Life and Work of a Public Health Crusader* (New York: Hill and Wang, 2003), p. 148.

9. E. Fuller, *Tinkers and Genius: The Story of the Yankee Inventors* (New York: Hastings House, 1955), pp. 205–6.

10. Ibid., pp. 174–77.

11. Roe, p. 126.

12. A. Hoffer and H. Osmond, "Treatment of Schizophrenia with Nicotinic Acid: A Ten Year Follow-up," *Acta Psychiatrica Scandinavica* 40 (1964): 171–89.

13. H. Osmond and A. Hoffer, "Massive Niacin Treatment in Schizophrenia: Review of a Nine-Year Study" *Lancet* 1 (1962): 316–19.

14. T. A. Ban and H. E. Lehmann, "Nicotinic Acid in the Treatment of Schizophrenias. Canadian Mental Health Association Collaborative Study Progress Report II," *Canadian Psychiatric Association Journal* 20 (1975): 103–12.

15. J. R. Wittenborn, E. S. P. Weber, and M. Brown, "Niacin in the Long-Term Treatment of Schizophrenia," *Archives of General Psychiatry* 28 (1973): 308–15.

16. R. Altschul, A. Hoffer, and J. D. Stephen, "Influence of Nicotinic Acid on Serum Cholesterol in Man," *Archives of Biochemistry and Biophysics* 54 (1955): 558–59.

CHAPTER 4

1. E. H. Reynolds, "Benefits and Risks of Folic Acid to the Nervous System," *Journal of Neurology, Neurosurgery, and Psychiatry* 72 (2002): 567–71.

2. M. Wintrobe, *Hematology, the Blossoming of a Science: A Story of Inspiration and Effort* (Philadelphia: Lea and Febiger, 1985), p. 65.

3. R. Hager, *The Life of Linus Pauling* (New York: Simon & Schuster, 1995), p. 36.

4. M. Wintrobe, *Hematology, the Blossoming of a Science: A Story of Inspiration and Effort* (Philadelphia: Lea and Febiger, 1985), pp. 219–20.

5. G. Ferry, *Dorothy Hodgkin. A Life* (Cold Spring Harbor, NY: Cold Spring Harbor Laboratory Press, 1998), p. 30.

6. Ibid., pp. 38–39.

7. Ibid., pp. 60–61.

8. S. B. McGrayne, *Nobel Prize Women in Science* (Secaucus, NJ: Birch Lane Press Book, 1998), p. 246.

9. Ferry, p. 259.

10. S. Van Tonder, J. Metz, and R. Green, "Vitamin B12 Metabolism in the Fruit Bat (*Rousettus aegyptiacus*). The Induction of Vitamin B12 Deficiency and Its Effect on Folate Levels," *British Journal of Nutrition* 34 (1975): 397–410.

11. A. D. M. Smith, "Megaloblastic Madness," *British Medical Journal* (1960): 1840–45.

12. Reynolds.

Chapter 5

1. S. Alderley, *The First Voyage Round the World by Magellan.* London: Hakluyt Society. 1874, Vol 52, p. 64, quoted in A. M. Beeuwkes, "The Prevalence of Scurvy Among Voyageurs to America—1493–1600." In A. M. Beeuwkes, E. N. Todhunter, and E. S. Weigley, eds. *Essays on History of Nutrition and Dietetics* (Chicago: The American Dietetic Association, 1967), pp. 88–91.

2. J. Cartier, *The Voyages of Jacques Cartier.* H. P. Biggar, trans-ed. Ottawa: Publications of the Public Archives of Canada No. 11, 1924, p. 204, quoted in A. M. Beeuwkes, "The Prevalence of Scurvy Among Voyageurs to America—1493–1600." In A. M. Beeuwkes, E. N. Todhunter, and E. S. Weigley, eds. *Essays on History of Nutrition and Dietetics* (Chicago: The American Dietetic Association, 1967), pp. 88–91.

3. J. Lind, *A Treatise on the Scurvy, 1772. A Facsimile of the Third Edition* (Birmingham AL: Classics of Medicine Library, 1980), p. 526.

4. J. C. Beaglehole, ed. *The Journals of Captain James Cook I. The Voyage of the Endeavour* (Cambridge: Hakluyt Society, 1955); quoted in K. J. Carpenter, *The History of Scurvy and Vitamin C* (Cambridge, UK: Cambridge University Press, 1986), p. 77.

5. T. Horwitz, *Blue Latitudes: Boldly Going Where Captain Cook Has Gone Before* (New York: Picador, 2002), p. 34.

6. S. R. Brown, *Scurvy. How a Surgeon, a Mariner, and a Gentleman Solved the Greatest Medical Mystery of the Age of Sail* (New York: Thomas Dunne Books, St. Martin's Griffin, 2003), p. 172.

7. K. J. Carpenter, *The History of Scurvy and Vitamin C* (Cambridge, UK: Cambridge University Press, 1986), p. 97.

8. C. Woodham-Smith, *Florence Nightingale* (New York: McGraw-Hill Book Company, 1951), p. 134.

9. L. F. Cooper, "Florence Nightingale's Contribution to Dietetics," in A. M. Beeuwkes, E. N. Todhunter, and E. S. Weigley, eds. *Essays on History of Nutrition and Dietetics* (Chicago: The American Dietetic Association, 1967), pp. 5–11.

10. P. Berton, *Arctic Grail. The Quest for the Northwest Passage and the North Pole, 1818–1909* (New York: Lyons Press, 2000), pp. 57–58.

11. Ibid, p. 146.

12. Carpenter, p. 236.

CHAPTER 6

1. K. Rajakumar, "Vitamin D, Cod-liver Oil, Sunlight, and Rickets: A Historical Perspective," *Pediatrics* 112 (2003): e132–e135.

2. P. De Kruif, *Hunger Fighters* (Rahway, NJ: Harcourt, Brace and Company, Inc., 1928), pp. 310–11.

3. M. F. Holick, "Vitamin D Deficiency," *New England Journal of Medicine* 357 (2007): 266–81.

CHAPTER 7

1. L. Bickel, *Mawson's Will. The Greatest Polar Survival Story Ever Written* (South Royalton, VT: Steerforth Press, 2000).

2. K. Michaelsson, H. Lithell, B. Vessby, et al., "Serum Retinol Levels and the Risk of Fracture," *New England Journal of Medicine* 348 (2003): 287–94.

3. J. D. Bremner, N. Fani, A. Ashraf, et al., "Functional Brain Imaging Alterations in Acne Patients Treated with Isotretinoin," *American Journal of Psychiatry* 162 (2005): 983–91.

4. M. F. Holick and M. Jenkins, *The UV Advantage* (United States of America: ibooks, 2003).

GLOSSARY

Absorb To take in. Nutrients are absorbed in the **gastrointestinal tract**.

Alpha helix The structure of **amino acid** chains in some **proteins.** This helix is stable and flexible and was first described by Linus Pauling. **Collagen** has an alpha helical structure.

Amine Organic compound containing nitrogen, found in **amino acids** and some vitamins.

Amino acid Chemical unit or building block that makes up **proteins.** We produce or synthesize some amino acids ourselves but need to have "essential" amino acids in our diet. **Tryptophan** is an essential amino acid.

Anemia Disorder of too few or poorly functioning red blood **cells.**

Ascorbic acid Vitamin C.

Autoimmune disease The immune system defends the body against foreign invaders such as bacteria, fungi, and viruses. Sometimes, the immune system treats part of the body as a foreign substance and attacks these parts. Common autoimmune illnesses include diabetes mellitus, thyroid illnesses, and rheumatoid arthritis. **Pernicious anemia** is an autoimmune illness in which there are antibodies against the **cells** that make **intrinsic** factor and against **intrinsic** factor itself.

Beriberi Deficiency disease caused by lack of Vitamin B1.

Calciferol Vitamin D2.

Calcitriol The biologically active form of Vitamin D formed in the kidney. The chemical name is 1,25-dihydroxycholecalciferol.

Capillary Small blood vessel. In **scurvy**, the **collagen** in capillary vessels is damaged and blood leaks out.

Carbohydrate An organic substance made up of carbon, oxygen, and hydrogen; an energy source. Produced during **photosynthesis** in plants. Sugar, or glucose, is a common carbohydrate.

Carotenoid Brightly colored pigment that aids in **photosynthesis.** Beta carotene, a carotenoid, is a precursor of Vitamin A.

Cartilage Type of connective **tissue** made up of **cells**, **collagen** fibers, and a solid, flexible **matrix.** Found in ears, the nose, and joints.

Cell Smallest unit of living organisms. Some microorganisms, such as bacteria, consist only of one cell. Humans consist of about one hundred trillion cells that are organized into **tissues.** Each cell is surrounded by a **cell membrane.**

Cell membrane The layer of **molecules** surrounding each **cell** that separates the outside of the **cell** from the inside. It is composed in part of **lipids,** such as **sterols.**

Cell nucleus The central part of the **cell** that contains the **chromosome.**

Chlorophyll Green pigment in plants that captures the energy from sunlight in **photosynthesis.** Similar in structure to **heme** and Vitamin B12.

Cholecalciferol Vitamin D3.

Cholesterol A **sterol molecule**, part of all **cell membranes.** A cholesterol-like **molecule**, 7-dehydrocholesterol, is the building block for **hormones** such as estrogen, testosterone, and Vitamin D.

Chromosome The structure made up of **DNA** and **proteins** that contains all our genetic material.

Cobalamin (or cyanocobalamin) Vitamin B12.

Collagen Common **helical protein** fiber found in the extracellular **matrix** of **connective tissues.** Found in skin, bone, teeth, tendons, muscles, and **capillary** walls. Damaged in **scurvy.**

Connective tissue **Tissue** including blood, bone, and **cartilage** that holds other structures together or, in the case of blood, connects them. Connective tissues consist of a **matrix** that contains **cells.**

Cornea The transparent dome over the iris and pupil of the eye that allows light into the back of the eye and focuses it.

7-dehydrocholesterol Provitamin D3. Found in the skin of animals.

Diffraction Breaking up of waves when they hit an object.

DNA Deoxyribonucleic acid, which carries genetic information in the **chromosome.**

Enrichment Restoration of mineral and vitamin losses caused by food processing or storage.

Enzyme A **protein** that increases the rate of a chemical reaction.

Epithelium A group of **cells,** or **tissue,** that covers the body surface and lines internal cavities, tubes, and organs. Skin is an epithelial **tissue.**

Ergocalciferol Vitamin D2.

Ergosterol A **sterol** molecule found in plants and yeasts. It is converted into Vitamin D when irradiated by **ultraviolet B radiation.**

Extrinsic factor Vitamin B12.

Folate Vitamin B9.

Fortification Addition of nutrients in excess of natural quantities found in food.

Gastrointestinal tract The tube in which food is digested, **absorbed,** and then excreted. It begins with the mouth, leads to the esophagus, and extends through the stomach and the small and large intestines, to end at the anus.

Gene A sequence of **DNA,** on the **chromosome,** which carries information about how to build **proteins.**

Helix Right- or left-handed curve in three dimensions. Springs are helical.

Heme Complex **protein** that carries iron, which in turn binds to oxygen in hemoglobin. Similar in structure to **chlorophyll** and Vitamin B12.

Histology Study of **tissues** and their structure.

Hormone Substance produced by one body **tissue** and released into the blood that affects the activity of another **tissue.** Insulin is a well-known hormone. Vitamins A and D have hormone-like actions.

Intrinsic factor Large **protein** made in the stomach to bind to Vitamin B12.

Lipid Fats, used as energy source and as components of **cell membranes.**

Macrocytic or megaloblastic anemia Anemia in which the red blood **cells** or their precursors in the bone marrow are larger than normal.

Matrix Substance in **connective tissues**, such as blood, bone, or **cartilage**, containing living **cells.** The matrix of blood is fluid, of bone is mineralized and hard, and of cartilage is gel-like.

Melanin Pigment in the skin that gives skin and hair their color and that absorbs **ultraviolet radiation.**

Metabolism The chemical reactions in the body responsible for growth, reproduction, and maintenance of structures.

Molecule Smallest part of a substance that has its qualities, made up of atoms.

Nanometer One billionth of a meter. Visible light has a wavelength of 400–700 nm. **Ultraviolet B radiation** has a wavelength of 280–315 nm. X-rays used in crystallography have a wavelength of .01–10 nm.

Neural tube defect A common birth defect in which the embryonic spinal tube does not close properly. **Folate** supplementation of grains and cereals in the United States makes this defect less common.

Niacin (or nicotinic acid) Vitamin B3.

Organ Group of **tissues.** For example, the heart, an organ, is made up of muscle **tissue** and blood and nerves.

Osteomalacia Softening of bones in adults. The bones are inadequately mineralized. Similar to **rickets** in children.

Osteoporosis This disease is common in postmenopausal women and is associated with fractures. Bone is adequately mineralized but broken down faster than it is rebuilt.

Pellagra Vitamin B3 deficiency disease. Features include the four Ds: dermatitis, diarrhea, dementia, and death.

Pernicious anemia Autoimmune disease in which the body does not **absorb** Vitamin B12.

Photosynthesis A metabolic pathway in plants by which carbon dioxide and water, using energy from sunlight, are changed to oxygen and **carbohydrates.**

Polyneuritis Inflammation of several nerves.

Protein Complex organic **molecule**, made of **amino acids.** It can be a structural component or **enzyme.**

Retinol Vitamin A.

Rickets Disease of children in which bones do not harden because of Vitamin D deficiency.

Rumen Part of the stomach in some animals. The food is partially digested in the rumen and then returned to the mouth, as a cud, for more chewing.

Scurvy Disease of disordered **collagen** because of Vitamin C deficiency.

Sterol A type of **lipid**, a component of the **cell membrane.** In animals, the best known sterol is **cholesterol.**

Thiamine Vitamin B1.

Tissue Group of similar **cells** that performs one function. **Epithelium** and muscle are examples of tissues. Tissues can form **organs.**

Tryptophan An essential **amino acid**, discovered by Sir Frederick Hopkins in 1901. It can be converted into the vitamin **niacin.** It is found in eggs, cod, cheese, milk, meat, and peanuts. Corn has very little tryptophan.

Ultraviolet B radiation Electromagnetic radiation from the sun of 280–315-nm length. This invisible radiation stimulates production of Vitamin D and leads to sun-tan, sunburn, and some skin cancers.

Xerophthalmia Extreme dryness of the eye that can lead to blindness.

BIBLIOGRAPHY

Altman, L. K. *The Story of Self-Experimentation in Medicine. Who Goes First?* New York: Random House, 1987.

Altschul, R., A. Hoffer, and J. D. Stephen, "Influence of Nicotinic Acid on Serum Cholesterol in Man," *Archives of Biochemistry and Biophysics* 54 (1955): 558–59.

Apple, R. D. *Vitamania. Vitamins in American Culture.* New Brunswick, NJ: Rutgers University Press, 1996.

Backstrand, J. R. "The History and Future of Food Fortification in the United States: A Public Health Perspective," *Nutrition Reviews* 60 (2002): 15–26.

Baldessarini, R. J., G. Stramentinoli, and J. F. Lipinski, "Methylation Hypothesis," *Archives of General Psychiatry* 36 (1979): 303–7.

Ban, T. A., and H. E. Lehmann, "Nicotinic Acid in the Treatment of Schizophrenias. Canadian Mental Health Association Collaborative Study Progress Report II," *Canadian Psychiatric Association Journal* 20 (1975): 103–12.

Barclay, A. J., A. Foster, and A. Sommer, "Vitamin A Supplements and Mortality Related to Measles: A Randomised Clinical Trial." *British Medical Journal (Clinical Research Ed.)* 294 (1987): 294–96.

Beeuwkes, A. M. "The Prevalence of Scurvy among Voyageurs to America—1493–1600," in A. M. Beeuwkes, E. N. Todhunter, and E. S. Weigley, eds. *Essays on History of Nutrition and Dietetics.* Chicago: The American Dietetic Association, 1967, 88–91.

Beeuwkes, A. M., E. N. Todhunter, and E. S. Weigley, eds., *Essays on History of Nutrition and Dietetics.* Chicago: The American Dietetic Association, 1967.

Berton, P., *Arctic Grail. The Quest for the Northwest Passage and the North Pole, 1818–1909.* New York: Lyons Press, 2000.

Bickel, L. *Mawson's Will. The Greatest Polar Survival Story Ever Written.* South Royalton, VT: Steerforth Press, 2000.

Bollet, A. J. *Plagues and Poxes. The Impact of Human History on Epidemic Disease.* New York: Demos, 2004.

Bremner, J. D., N. Fani, A. Ashraf, et al., "Functional Brain Imaging Alterations in Acne Patients Treated with Isotretinoin," *The American Journal of Psychiatry* 162 (2005): 983–91.

Brown, S. R. *Scurvy. How a Surgeon, a Mariner, and a Gentleman Solved the Greatest Medical Mystery of the Age of Sail*. New York: Thomas Dunne Books, St. Martin's Griffin, 2003.

Burgess, R. C. "Deficiency Diseases in Prisoners-of-War at Changi, Singapore," *Lancet* 2 (1946): 411–18.

Campbell, K. A. "Knots in the Fabric: Richard Pearson Strong and the Bilibid Prison Vaccine Trials, 1905–1906," *Bulletin of the History of Medicine* 68 (1994): 600–38.

Carpenter, K. J. *The History of Scurvy and Vitamin C*. Cambridge, UK: Cambridge University Press, 1986.

Carpenter, K. J. "Forgotten Mysteries in the Early History of Vitamin D," *The Journal of Nutrition* 129 (1999): 923–27.

Carpenter, K. J. *Beriberi, White Rice, and Vitamin B. A Disease, A Cause, and A Cure*. Berkeley: University of California Press, 2000.

Carpenter, K. J. "Harriette Chick and the Problem of Rickets," *The Journal of Nutrition* 138 (2008): 827–32.

Chick, H. "Study of Rickets in Vienna 1919–22," *Medical History* 20 (1976): 41–51.

Cooper, L. F. "Florence Nightingale's Contribution to Dietetics," in A. M. Beeuwkes, E. N. Todhunter, and E. S. Weigley, eds. *Essays on History of Nutrition and Dietetics*. Chicago: The American Dietetic Association, 1967, 5–11.

De Kruif, P. *Hunger Fighters*. Rahway, NJ: Harcourt, Brace and Company, Inc., 1928.

Drew, L. R. and A. S. Truswell, "Wernicke's Encephalopathy and Thiamine Fortification of Food: Time for a New Direction?" *The Medical Journal of Australia* 168 (1998): 534–35.

Dunn, P. M. "Professor Armand Trousseau (1801–67) and the Treatment of Rickets," *Archives of Disease in Childhood. Fetal and Neonatal Edition* 80 (1999): F155–F157.

Ellison, J. B. "Intensive Vitamin Therapy in Measles," *British Medical Journal* 2 (1932): 708–11.

Etheridge, E. W. *The Butterfly Caste: A Social History of Pellagra in the South*. Westport, CT: Greenwood, 1972.

Fee, E. *Disease and Discovery. A History of the Johns Hopkins School of Hygiene and Public Health, 1916–1939*. Baltimore, MD: The Johns Hopkins University Press, 1987.

Ferry, G. *Dorothy Hodgkin. A Life*. Cold Spring Harbor, NY: Cold Spring Harbor Laboratory Press, 1998.

Fuller, E. *Tinkers and Genius: The Story of the Yankee Inventors*. New York: Hastings House, 1955.

Funk, C. *The Vitamines*. Authorized Translation from Second German Edition. Baltimore, MD: Williams and Wilkins Company, 1922.

Gratzer, W. *Terrors of the Table: The Curious History of Nutrition*. Oxford, UK: Oxford University Press, 2005.

Hager, R. *The Life of Linus Pauling*. New York: Simon & Schuster, 1995.

Hardy, A. "Beriberi, Vitamin B1, and World Food Policy," *Medical History* 39 (1995): 61–77.

Hoffer, A., and H. Osmond, "Treatment of Schizophrenia with Nicotinic Acid: A Ten Year Follow-up," *Acta Psychiatrica Scandinavica* 40 (1964): 171–89.

Holick, M. F. "Sunlight and Vitamin D for Bone Health and Prevention of Auto-immune Diseases, Cancers, and Cardiovascular Disease," *The American Journal of Clinical Nutrition* 80 (suppl.) (2004): 1678S–1688S.

Holick, M. F. "Vitamin D Deficiency," *New England Journal of Medicine* 357 (2007): 266–81.

Holick, M. F., and M. Jenkins, *The UV Advantage*. New York: ibooks, Incorporated, 2003.

Horwitz, T. *Blue Latitudes: Boldly Going Where Captain Cook Has Gone Before*. New York: Picador, 2002.

Klawans, H. *Newton's Madness. Further Tales of Clinical Neurology*. New York: Harper & Row, 1990.

Kraut, A. M. *Goldberger's War: The Life and Work of a Public Health Crusader*. New York: Hill and Wang, 2003.

Lederer, S. E. *Subjected to Science. Human Experimentation in America before the Second World War*. Baltimore, MD: The Johns Hopkins University Press, 1997.

Lehrer, S. *Explorers of the Body*. New York: Doubleday & Company, 1979.

Lind, J. *A Treatise on the Scurvy, 1772. A Facsimile of the Third Edition*. Birmingham, AL: Classics of Medicine Library, 1980.

McCollum, E. V. *From Kansas Farm Boy to Scientist*. Lawrence, KS: University of Kansas Press, 1964.

McCollum, E. V., and J. E. Becker, *Food, Nutrition and Health*, 6th ed. Baltimore, MD: The Lord Baltimore Press, 1947.

McCollum, E. V. and N. Simmonds, *The Newer Knowledge of Nutrition*. New York: The Macmillan Company, 1927.

McGee, H. *On Food and Cooking: The Science and Lore of the Kitchen*. New York: Collier Books, Macmillan Publishing Company, 1984.

McGrayne, S. B. *Nobel Prize Women in Science*. Secaucus, NJ: Birch Lane Press Book, 1998.

Michaelsson, K., H. Lithell, B. Vessby, et al., "Serum Retinol Levels and the Risk of Fracture," *New England Journal of Medicine* 348 (2003): 287–94.

Osmond, H., and A. Hoffer, "Massive Niacin Treatment in Schizophrenia: Review of a Nine-Year Study," *Lancet* 1 (1962): 316–19.

Pauling, L. "Orthomolecular Psychiatry: Varying the Concentrations of Substances Normally Present in the Human Body May Control Mental Disease," *Science* 160 (1968): 265–71.

Rajakumar, K. "Infantile Scurvy: A Historical Perspective," *Pediatrics* 108 (2001): e76–e78.

Rajakumar, K. "Vitamin D, Cod-Liver Oil, Sunlight, and Rickets: A Historical Perspective," *Pediatrics* 112 (2003): e132–e135.

Rajakumar, K., S. L. Greenspan, S. B. Thomas, and M. F. Holick. "Solar Ultraviolet Radiation and Vitamin D: A Historical Perspective," *American Journal of Public Health* 97 (2007): 1746–54.

Rajakumar, K., and S. B. Thomas, "Reemerging Nutritional Rickets. A Historical Perspective," *Archives of Pediatrics & Adolescent Medicine* 159 (2005): 335–41.

Reuler, J. B., D. E. Girard, and T. G. Cooney, "Wernicke's Encephalopathy," *New England Journal of Medicine* 1038 (1985): 1035–39.

Reynolds, E. H. "Benefits and Risks of Folic Acid to the Nervous System," *Journal of Neurology, Neurosurgery, and Psychiatry* 72 (2002): 567–71.

Rider, A. A., and Elmer Verner McCollum, "A Biographical Sketch," *The Journal of Nutrition* 100 (1970): 1–10.

Roe, D. A. *A Plague of Corn. The Social History of Pellagra.* Ithaca, NY: Cornell University Press, 1973.

Roe, D. A. "Lucy Wills (1888–1964): A Biographical Sketch," *The Journal of Nutrition* 108 (1978): 1379–83.

Semba, R. D. "Vitamin A as "Anti-Infective" Therapy. 1920–1940," *The Journal of Nutrition* 129 (1999): 783–91.

Smith, A. D. M. "Megaloblastic Madness," *British Medical Journal* (1960): 1840–1845.

Sommer, A. "A Bridge Too Near," in *The Progress of Nations.* New York: UNICEF, 1995: 10–11.

Sommer, A., and K. West, *Vitamin A Deficiency. Health, Survival, and Vision.* New York: Oxford University Press, 1996.

Strey, G. "Wisconsin's Fight over the Demon Spread," *Wisconsin Magazine of History* (Autumn 2001): 3–15.

Swazey, J. P., and K. Reeds, *Today's Medicine, Tomorrow's Science. Essays on Paths of Discovery in the Biomedical Sciences.* Washington, DC: U.S. Department of Health, Education, and Welfare, 1978.

Van Tonder, S., J. Metz, and R. Green, "Vitamin B12 Metabolism in the Fruit Bat (*Rousettus aegyptiacus*). The Induction of Vitamin B12 Deficiency and Its Effect on Folate Levels," *The British Journal of Nutrition* 34 (1975): 397–410.

Victor, M., and P. I. Yakovlev, "S. S. Korsakoff's Psychic Disorder in Conjunction with Peripheral Neuritis. A Translation of Korsakoff's Original Article with Brief Comments on the Author and His Contributions to Clinical Medicine," *Neurology* 5 (1955): 394–406.

Wadsworth, G. R. "Tropical Macrocytic Anaemia: The Investigations of Lucy Wills in India," *Asia-Pacific Journal of Public Health* 2 (1988): 265–73.

Williams, R. R. *Toward the Conquest of Beriberi.* Cambridge, MA: Harvard University Press, 1961.

Williams, R. R., and T. D. Spies, *Vitamin B1 and Its Use in Medicine.* New York: The Macmillan Company, 1938.

Wilson, L. G. "The Clinical Definition of Scurvy and the Discovery of Vitamin C," *Journal of the History of Medicine and Allied Sciences* 30 (1975): 40–60.

Wintrobe, M. *Hematology, the Blossoming of a Science: A Story of Inspiration and Effort.* Philadelphia, PA: Lea and Febiger, 1985.

Wittenborn, J. R., E. S. P. Weber, and M. Brown, "Niacin in the Long-Term Treatment of Schizophrenia," *Archives of General Psychiatry* 28 (1973): 308–15.

Wolf, G. "M. Mori's Definitive Recognition of Vitamin A Deficiency and Its Cure in Children," *Nutrition* 14 (1998): 481–84.

Wolf, G. "The Discovery of Vitamin D: The Contribution of Adolf Windaus," *The Journal of Nutrition* 134 (2004): 1299–1302.

Woodham-Smith, C., *Florence Nightingale.* New York: McGraw-Hill Book Company, 1951.

INDEX

About the Author

FRANCES RACHEL FRANKENBURG, M.D., is Associate Professor of Psychiatry at Boston University School of Medicine and Adjunct Clinical Professor at Massachusetts College of Pharmacy and Health Sciences. She is also Chief of Inpatient Psychiatry, and Director of Medical Student Education, at the Edith Nourse Rogers Memorial Veterans Administration Medical Center at Bedford, MA. In addition, Frankenburg is Associate Director at the McLean Hospital Laboratory for the Study of Adult Development. She has written numerous articles for academic journals, and is a reviewer for multiple journals, including *New England Journal of Medicine, Archives of General Psychiatry, Harvard Review of Psychiatry,* and *International Journal of Geriatric Psychiatry.* Her many awards include the National Alliance for the Mentally Ill Exemplary Psychiatrist Award.

About the Series Editor

JULIE SILVER, M.D., is Assistant Professor, Harvard Medical School, Department of Physical Medicine and Rehabilitation, and is on the medical staff at Brigham & Women's, Massachusetts General, and Spaulding Rehabilitation Hospitals in Boston, Massachusetts. Dr. Silver has authored, edited, or co-edited more than a dozen books, including medical textbooks and consumer health guides. She is also the Chief Editor of Books at Harvard Health Publications. Dr. Silver has won many awards, including the American Medical Writers Association Solimene Award for Excellence in Medical Writing and the prestigious Lane Adams Quality of Life Award from the American Cancer Society. Silver is active teaching health care providers how to write and publish, and she is the Founder and Director of an annual seminar facilitated by the Harvard Medical School Department of Continuing Education, "Publishing Books, Memoirs and Other Creative Non-Fiction."

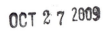